Autophagy

Discover How to Live Healthy and Longer with Your Self-Cleansing Body's Natural Intelligence. Start a Fasting Diet Activating the Anti-Aging Process to Lose Weight Safely

Written By

Rachel Dash

By reading this document, the reader agrees that under no circumstances is the author responsible for any losses, direct or indirect, which are incurred as a result of the use of information contained within this document, including, but not limited to, — errors, omissions, or inaccuracies.

Table of Contents

Introduction

Thank you for purchasing *Autophagy: Discover How to Live Healthy and Longer with Your Self-Cleansing Body's Natural Intelligence.* In this book, you will learn about Autophagy and all of the health benefits that it has to offer. These benefits are numerous and include weight loss, increased energy, improved immune system functioning, and cancer-fighting ability. Yet the good things autophagy can do for you extend far beyond these and they will be explored specifically in order to help you better understand how you can improve your life by tapping into this important and natural cellular process. It is not as difficult as you might think.

Autophagy has become a buzz word in the health and fitness industry, much like the Atkins Diet and Keto. Like many other buzz words, autophagy is a term that many people are exposed to but relatively few understand. Autophagy is generally thought of as being similar to the more familiar apoptosis, which many will have learned about in school. But autophagy is quite from different this other major form of cell death, and it is this difference that will help you improve your health and wellbeing with this pathway. As you will discover, intermittent fasting, water fasting, fasting-mimicking, and other diets can stimulate autophagy and, as a result, lead to improved health outcomes and longevity.

Autophagy is how the body engages in the survival of the fittest on a cellular level. Autophagy allows the human body to consume and recycle components for a variety of purposes. These components can be used to build new cells or for energy. This process can be activated in many different ways, of which among the more common is through a protein called AMP-activated protein kinase, or AMPK. AMP Kinase is, in fact, an enzyme that plays an important role in energy conservation and homeostasis in the human body.

AMP Kinase is generated in situations when the body needs to metabolize its own components for energy, as is the case when you are fasting both intentionally or simply because it is early in the day and you have not eaten yet. This is an important concept that will be explored in the book. Fasting can be something that you do deliberately over a long period, or it can be incorporated into periods in your day as part of a periodic fasting regime (i.e. intermittent fasting). As you will discover, many processes or foods can be used to stimulate autophagy for beneficial reasons.

For instance, much research has focused on foods that can play a role in stimulating autophagy for the purposes of fighting cancer or discouraging diseases. Many men and women choose to incorporate these types of foods into their diets even though they are not facing the ravages of cancer or another serious disease. The Reishi mushroom has been studied because of the role it plays in the suppression of colon cancer cell growth through the phosphorylation of a version of AMP Kinase. Green tea and ginger have also been studied because of their proven effects in cancer suppression by way of compounds EGCG and 6-Shagaal, respectively.

The human body does not really distinguish between fasting and starvation. Part of the reason why fasting works so well in stimulating autophagy is that the human body is always preparing for the worst. If you have not eaten for a prolonged period, your body realizes that it does not make sense to waste energy and other resources on components that are not contributing to the overall survival of the organism. This allows the body to use fasting, exercise and even reduced oxygen as triggers for autophagy. Stimulating autophagy, therefore, is nothing more than taking advantage of how your body has evolved to deal with stress and to survive.

Stimulation of autophagy, or Autophagy as it is conceptualized in this book, requires an understanding of what autophagy is and why it is. Autophagy is a type of cell death, and it is critical for it to be distinguished from the better-known apoptosis. Apoptosis is programmed cell death, which makes autophagy a form of non-programmed cell death. This has led to some perceiving autophagy as a haphazard process that represents sort of a "blue screen of death" for the body's cells, but nothing could be further from the truth.

Autophagy is how the body streamlines itself, a concept that will be further explored in the first two chapters. When we speak of survival of the fittest in the context of autophagy, what we mean is that sometimes the body finds it necessary to remove some components and encourage others. This happens on a molecular and cellular level through processes like autophagy. Autophagy allows the body to acutely and in a highly-controlled fashion remove cells that no longer align with the body's needs.

This sort of process can be essential to the survival of an organism, which is a major reason why autophagy has evolved to become a normal process in humans. Indeed, one of the goals of this book is to teach you how you can use this natural process of the body to lose weight, target fat, reduce your chances of cancer or other health ailments, and improve your wellbeing. Autophagy (as well as the specific processes that fall under its scope) is not a fad diet. This is a scientifically proven, normal process whose study has resulted in the awarding of a Nobel Prize (the most recent of which was in 2016).

Why is autophagy significant enough to award a scientist a Nobel Prize for its study? Research has found that doctors can use compounds isolated from plants to stimulate autophagy against cancer cells. Cancer is by definition the unregulated and dysfunctional growth of cells and tissues that eventually leads to death. Cancer cells cause damage to the organs where they form. Cancer cells eventually metastasize (or spread) to other tissues, leading to organ failure and eventual demise. Cell death is how the human body normally deals with dysfunctional cells. In particular, autophagy is the process that would allow the body to acutely remove cellular components through activation or up-regulation of proteins like AMP Kinase. The body's ultimate goal is to remove cells before they become cancerous, but no one is perfect and sometimes our bodies fail in this pursuit.

If scientists can tap into autophagy in states of cancer, then they may be able to reverse the cancer growth (or destroy the cells) without risking damaging normal tissues as happens with chemotherapy and radiation therapy. These types of treatments are regarded with fear by many because of the symptoms and side effects that stem from damage to normal cells during the attempt to eradicate the abnormal ones. But by tapping into natural autophagy processes, the human body would be able to breakdown these cancerous growths in an organized and systematic fashion without affecting the body's normal machinery.

This is part of what distinguishes autophagy from apoptosis, an important distinction that will be detailed at length in this book. This is a critical line to draw in your head because co-opting Autophagy will allow you to live a healthy and vigorous life, free from obesity and disease, while apoptosis would represent premature death of tissues. It may help to remember the word premature in the context of apoptosis as this will allow you to distinguish it from autophagy which is generally not premature, but ordered and necessary.

Because autophagy is thrown around so much on the internet, it is important to have a deep understanding of what it is on both the cellular and tissue level, which will be accomplished in the first and second chapters. Because of how autophagy works to recycle and remove redundant or problematic cellular components, the uses and advantages of autophagy tend to focus on certain areas. Autophagy can be used to reduce inflammation, stimulate anti-aging effects, improve immune function, improve brain function, provide protection from neurodegenerative diseases, and help men and women to avoid cancer. Indeed, it has been demonstrated that a 7-day fast once a year can be used to completely remove cancer cells from the body.

Part of what makes autophagy so powerful is that it operates on a molecular and cellular level, and can even be used to reshape tissues. This aspect of autophagy - that it works on a minute level to efface great changes - may give the discussion of autophagy the impression of a broken record, but it pervades all aspects of the autophagy picture. For instance, fasting and high-intensity interval training (or HIIT) can so dramatically improve health because the minute changes that they cause can lead to large "macro" effects on the body's organs and systems.

Like other health and fitness buzz words, autophagy is used enough that it what it actually means can become obscured. In the first chapter, the reader will be provided with a working definition of autophagy, one that begins to explore the different types of autophagy (which will be examined further in later chapters). The reader will also partake in a discussion on why autophagy works, which will help to draw a thick dividing line between autophagy, apoptosis, and the general concept of cell death.

The benefits of autophagy are extensive enough that books can be (and have been) written on the subject. Indeed, it has been argued that the longevity that we see in certain parts of the world like Japan and Greece can actually be attributed to foods and eating regimens that stimulate autophagy in various ways. It seems to be the case that these areas of the long, continuous settlement have preserved secrets from the very distant past. The major benefits of autophagy include anti-cancer and anti-aging effects, but as the reader has already seen, the benefits do not end there. These benefits will be explored in the second chapter.

The question of how autophagy works is another area upon which books have been written. There are many subtopics within that subject alone. Indeed, this is an area that continues to receive research funding internationally as more is learned about the many ways non-programmed cell death can be stimulated or halted. Cancer cells can prevent the human body from accomplishing apoptosis or autophagy while stimulating autophagy with food, drugs, or dieting can fight cancer and confer other advantages. This note underlies the discussion of how autophagy works, and all of this will be detailed in the third chapter.

There are many ways to stimulate autophagy, some of which the reader will already be familiar with. Intermittent fasting is a popular type of eating regime that has found many supporters in the health and fitness community. Intermittent fasting can allow the man or woman trying it to remove fat while preserving muscle. It does this by actually tapping into how human beings consume food and fast naturally.

Indeed, many modern men and women in the Western world take for granted the wide availability of food that characterizes most Western countries. Your ancestor's thousands of years ago did not have refrigerators, freezers, and pantries to store food year-round so that they might eat at all hours of the day. They would rise early in the morning to hunt and fish, and then they would have to skin and cook their quarry, which meant that they may not eat until noontime or later. This meant that they would have been fasting from their last meal the day before until they were able to eat the meal that they had just prepared. As groundbreaking and powerful as intermittent fasting is, it merely represents a more natural state of living for human beings. Fasting and other ways to stimulate autophagy will be explored in the fourth chapter.

These other methods of stimulating autophagy include water fasting and other prolonged fasting diets. Extended water fasting has become a powerful way for many men and women to incorporate autophagy stimulation into their daily lives. Although some regard extended water fasting as difficult, the benefits that it can lead to by stimulating autophagy are clear. Diets that involve stimulating ketosis (the creation of ketone bodies) in the body will also be examined along with water fasting in the fifth chapter.

Among the most powerful cohorts of supporters of Autophagy as a process men and women can incorporate into their lives are the health and fitness community. Men and women bodybuilders and fitness enthusiasts can all find ways to incorporate autophagy into their lives as a way of losing fat and preserving muscle. Intermittent fasting is the most obvious way of accomplishing this. Intermittent fasting is generally divided into two types: alternate-day fasting and time-restricted feeding. In the sixth chapter, we will explore how diets that involve autophagy, such as intermittent fasting, can be incorporated into your workout regimen to improve your results.

As we have seen, autophagy can be rapidly and reliably stimulated with food. When one is dieting, it is easy to get into the mindset that food equals bad, but this is not necessarily true.

Indeed, this is a type of thinking that must be broken if you truly want to benefit from Autophagy. Most people know that oatmeal first thing in the morning can raise metabolism and lead to fat loss. Well, many foods do basically the same thing but through autophagy. The many foods that can stimulate autophagy will be explored in the seventh chapter.

Fasting is the best way to stimulate autophagy because this period of fast encourages the body to work toward recycling components and improving homeostasis. Most programs that stimulate autophagy involve fasting of some form of another, including the limited type of fasting known as intermittent fasting. But there are other diets that tap into the importance of fasting without actually fasting. The fasting-mimicking diet is just such a diet, and it will be explored along with related topics in fasting in the eighth chapter.

Autophagy is technical enough that most people do not truly understand it and a few dedicate their careers to studying it. In the ninth chapter, the reader will learn tips to help them with stimulating autophagy through fasting. Some want help in fasting for days and days, while others want tips on how to get the most from intermittent fasting. All of the fasting tips you need to get started on your forays into fasting will be explored in the ninth chapter.

Stimulating autophagy is complex, but that does not mean that you and others like you cannot do it. Indeed, it can be said that the autophagy processes are complex, but the stimulation that you can do externally is easy. It may be as simple as not eating for eighteen hours or drinking more water than usual. In the tenth chapter, you will learn how you can stimulate and optimize autophagy by incorporating autophagy secrets and tips into your life.

Autophagy is not a mere fad. Autophagy has been shown to reduce the risk of cancer and lengthen life. Indeed, if autophagy were a drug it would probably be too expensive for you to afford it. Fortunately for you, autophagy is not a drug. It is something that your body does naturally, but which process has been undermined by the Western tendency to overeat and introduce toxic chemicals into the body. *Autophagy: Discover How to Live Healthy and Longer with Your Self-Cleansing Body's Natural Intelligence* will help you to reverse this trend in your own life and improve your quality of life. It all begins with an in-depth exploration of what autophagy is and why it is.

Chapter 1: Understanding Autophagy

Health regimens that tap into the human body's natural methods of achieving homeostasis have become more popular in recent decades as men and women of divergent backgrounds attempt to connect with Mother Nature and all of her secrets. Diets like the Paleo Diet and Atkins all purport to represent more natural ways of eating and living, suppositions that are not always far from the truth. Indeed, assertions made by those who promote these diets, that our ancestors consumed foods high in proteins, fats, and fibers, but low in carbohydrates, these assertions have been supported by the historical record and by scientific discoveries about the body.

Much of the science surrounding Autophagy is based around just this approach: attempting to understand the body's natural way of recycling components and achieving equilibrium. In fact, autophagy can be understood as to how the body naturally achieves a balance between all of its and its needs. The necessity of this type of balance should be clear. Just as a large town or even a business requires a records department, police department, sanitation department, and the like, so too does the human body have to approach its functions from the standpoint of achieving a balance between often disparate goals and requirements.

Just as a large town has a need to remove redundant or unnecessary components, so too does a human body or even a cell. In fact, autophagy occurs at a cellular level: a process that is able to achieve macro or organism-level effects by building on the individual cell and tissue effects that begin often with a simple signal. Autophagy and other processes similar to it are stimulated by various factors that often compete with one another to lead to a result. If the factors in favor of autophagy outweigh those that are against it, than autophagy wins and the body begins to engage in a process that can lead to a number of benefits, which include weight loss, increased energy, the release of human growth hormone, anti-cancer effects, and anti-aging effects.

If the factors discouraging autophagy outweigh those activating or stimulating it, then autophagy is blocked on the cellular level. This often is the case in cancer, where cancer cells are able to release signaling molecules that phosphorylate or otherwise inhibit important protein or signaling molecules. Of course, this mechanism of cancer is not natural to our bodies but represents a dysfunctional error that can lead to death if doctors are not able to treat it. Fortunately, science has a solution here. By finding ways to stimulate autophagy, even in the context of cancer, we can often slow or even reverse the effects of cancer, which can lead to survival.

Studies of the genetics of autophagy are regarded as significant enough that they lead to an awarding of a Nobel Prize in 2016 to a Japanese scientist. Autophagy (and the dysfunctional cancer pathways that interfere with it) is coordinated by an intricate mélange of genes, proteins, signaling molecules, and competing pathways. Of course, this is the norm in the human body, allowing the body to achieve homeostasis by sort of a majority rules decision. As chaotic as it may seem, these types of pathways evolved because they work. Autophagy exists in us because it serves a purpose and does some good.

Autophagy, a type of non-apoptotic cell death, involves the consumption of cellular components by organelles as a result of a signaling pathway. Many different proteins and molecules play a role here, but the more important ones have been well-studied. Indeed, scientists now know enough about these molecules that they can research foods that stimulate them and determine whether claims about health benefits related to these foods have any basis in fact.

The results may come as a surprise to some. It has been shown that foods that activate or stimulate the important AMP-activated protein kinase (which itself stimulates autophagy) have been shown to reduce the risk of cancer, fight cancer, increase longevity, and confer a host of other positive health benefits. This dispels the beliefs of some that diets that purport to tap into more ancient ways of living (like Autophagy) are not based in science or are tantamount to wishful thinking.

Autophagy, the process of using the body's natural cellular autophagy process to confer health benefits, is anything but wishful thinking. In fact, autophagy is occurring in your body right now, and it most likely is acting to preserve your cells (and your body as a whole) from components that would eventually derail it. Think of autophagy as a natural and healthy type of recycling that occurs in your body. This healthy recycling is very far removed from those distorted beliefs about fasting and diet that some detractors spew. Learning more about autophagy, including gaining an in-depth understanding of what it is, may help in your attempts to incorporate this powerful tool into your daily life.

Autophagy Defined

Autophagy, or non-programmed cell death, is a process that is constantly occurring in cells and tissues in the body. Apoptosis occurs at the cellular level, which means that it takes place within the cell membrane through the action of several cell organelles, of which among the most important is arguably the autophagosome. This organelle fuses with the lysosome in autophagy. Autophagy can be defined as the process of cellular breakdown or recycling that occurs within the cell. Some also add to this definition that autophagy processes are able to use components broken down for fuel (hence recycling) with the help of the mitochondria.

The autophagosomes, lysosomes, endoplasmic reticula, mitochondria, and numerous other vesicles and smaller particles within the cell participate in autophagy. Autophagy stems from a Greek root and it means "self-eating." Many in the health and fitness community like to think of autophagy as the breakdown of no longer needed cellular components for energy, which is different from the programmed death or "suicide" of cells in apoptosis. Autophagy occurs on an as-needed basis as opposed to being pre-programmed like apoptosis. This allows autophagy to be upregulated or downregulated as needed, so there will always be cells undergoing autophagy somewhere.

The idea is to upregulate autophagy for the purposes of health and fitness benefits, which are often referred to as Autophagy. Metabolism is important in autophagy as your basal metabolic rate works in tandem with processes like autophagy to cause you to lose weight, maintain the same weight, or to perhaps gain weight. This all happens at the cellular level through the breakdown of components like fat particles in hepatic cells and other body tissues. Autophagy is capable of acting in cells of many different types in the body, which is how it is able to achieve the Autophagy results that most of you desire.

Indeed, autophagy even plays a role in upregulating T1 and T2 helper lymphocytes leading to a stronger immune response.

Autophagy is significant in helping the body fight disease processes and increasing longevity to such a degree that cancer cells attempt to disrupt the process as part of their disordered growth. But we are jumping the gun a little bit. Let us dive deeper into understanding how autophagy works at the cellular level.

Autophagy basically involves different types of phagocytosis that occur within the cell. Phagocytosis is another word that comes from the Greek, and it basically means "cell eating." This word refers to the ability of cells to consume components, generally those that originate outside the cell. As you will soon see, autophagy, although it takes place within the cell, can involve the digestion of components that came from outside of the cell (such as a recycled cell whose components need to be broken down). These components, such as amino acids, can be used to build new components or for energy.

Autophagy can be quite complex, which is why an entire chapter in this book is devoted to understanding how this process works. This process is carefully controlled by signaling processes in the body, but it can be stimulated (and manipulated) by things that we do, such as the activities we do with our body and what we put into our body.

Why Autophagy Works

Autophagy works because the body needs a way of breaking down its own components and using them as material for other cells and tissues, and for energy. Therefore, autophagy represents a way that nature has solved the problem of not generating waste that ultimately serves no purpose. Think about it this way, as human beings, we generate a ton of garbage that is tossed into garbage dumps, sewage sites, and perhaps ultimately makes its way into waterways and oceans. This is trash that serves no purpose after its original purpose is done as it is no longer being used for anything. What autophagy does is take in the body's garbage and recycle it so that only the things the body absolutely needs to get rid of are removed in the renal system and GI tract.

But autophagy is more than a mere way for the body to hold on to its recycling goodies. This process also allows the body to achieve a measure of homeostasis. Homeostasis is a fancy way of saying equilibrium, and all animals must maintain internal and external homeostasis or else they would become extinct. Autophagy is also a way for the body to produce those compounds or molecules that it needs, which is why this process is upregulated in periods of fasting or intense exercise, such as in high-intensity interval training (or HIIT).

This latter type of autophagy is the primary subject of this book. Here we will attempt to understand how men and women can use fasting, exercise, and food to tap into the body's own recycling system. This can allow you to achieve a host of goals, whether they are weight loss, increased immune function, anti-aging benefits, or anti-cancer benefits. The benefits of autophagy are numerous. They will be explored further in a later chapter, but we can introduce some of the functions of autophagy here by way of an introduction. Some of the roles that autophagy plays in the body include:

- Cell death
- Tumor suppression
- Repair of damaged cellular components
- Removal of infectious particles

Autophagy, unfortunately, is also a target for processes that seek to derail it, as we mentioned earlier. Autophagy experiences interference by infectious agents like bacterial proteins and viral particles. Autophagy is also interfered with by tumor cells, perhaps the most well-known type of interference. Tumor cells evolve ways to resist destruction by autophagy and apoptosis, and this often involves the synthesis of proteins and enzymes that interrupt the normal signaling pathway of autophagy. Some of these pathways will be explored in greater detail later.

Autophagy for Health

Most people reading this book are interested in the uses of autophagy for health benefits. You may have learned about autophagy on the internet or on social media, and you are interested in learning more. Some of the claims made about autophagy may seem outlandish. It has been purported that autophagy can have anti-cancer effects, anti-aging effects, and can boost the immune system. It has even been said that autophagy can increase human growth hormone release in the body and cause drastic weight loss. All of these claims are true.

Indeed, scientists have only tapped the iceberg when it comes to all of the powerful things that autophagy can do in the human body. It has been demonstrated that men and women living in places where they consume foods that stimulate autophagy like green tea, ginger, and other foods have been blessed with greater longevity, lower rates of cancer, and other indications of good health compared to other populations. Much study has been devoted to uncovering the secrets of these peoples, and one of the links in the chain may be autophagy.

Autophagy, as you have learned, is a natural body process that helps the human body in several caretaking activities, but it does much more than this. Some of the more significant effects and qualities of autophagy will be explored later, but for now, we can point out some of the more significant aspects. Benefits of autophagy include:

- Ability to fight cancer
- Ability to protect against neurodegenerative diseases, such as Parkinson's Disease
- Ability to regulate other cell organelles to enhance cellular function
- Ability to protect against misfolded proteins that can cause amyloid diseases

- Ability to improve neuroplasticity, brain function, and brain structure
- Ability to strengthen the immune system both directly and indirectly
- Enhancing the growth of cardiovascular cells
- Protecting against aging
- Protecting DNA from degradation
- Protecting the body's organs and tissues from damage

Autophagy is able to accomplish this through the numerous autophagy genes that lead to the release of proteins, enzymes, and signaling molecules that regulate autophagy and other cellular processes in a positive way. The awarding of a Nobel Prize to Yoshinori Ohsumi in 2016 was related to his study of autophagy-related genes, of which there are known to be at least 32. The study of these genes has allowed scientists to elucidate some of the mechanisms of autophagy.

Types of Autophagy (and Induction)

Several different types of autophagy are known, of which microautophagy, macroautophagy, and chaperone-mediated autophagy are the most important. The differences between these three will be explored later, but they will be summarized here. Macroautophagy is regarded as the main autophagy pathway. It involves the eradication of damaged proteins or organelles' using what is known as an autophagosome.

Autophagosomes fuse with the more well-known lysosome, which is then able to breakdown, the components.

Microautophagy involves the engulfment of particles by the lysosome directly, without the mediation of the autophagosome. This process generally occurs by invagination, or folding in, of the lysosome's membrane. Chaperone-mediated autophagy is the third major pathway, and it is still being actively studied. This pathway involves the formation of a protein complex and an intricate pattern of recognition. This process is distinct from other types of autophagy because of the specificity that is involved in stimulating it compared to the other types of autophagy.

Autophagy can be induced or stimulated in a variety of ways, all of which will be examined closely in this book. Fasting is one of the most reliable ways of stimulating autophagy, and it is recommended by health enthusiasts who have actively studied the best ways to activate this pathway. Fasting can take a variety of forms, including the well-known intermittent fasting, or so-called alternate day fasting, which involves punctuating days of fasting with "normal" days of eating. Dieting and exercise can also be used to predictably stimulate autophagy. The main ways of stimulating this pathway (that will be examined here) include:

- Fasting
- Dieting with the Ketogenic Diet (or similar regimens)

- Exercise, especially HIIT (high-intensity interval training)

In subsequent chapters, ways in which autophagy can be induced to help you achieve your health goals will be more closely examined. These goals may include weight loss, targeted fat loss, and increase in muscle mass and definition, but they may also include anti-aging benefits and cancer-protective effects. Indeed, many people who decide to fast do it not because they are attempting to align their appearance with their desired body image but because they are interested in living a long, healthy life. It is not necessary to isolate a single goal when it comes to integrating autophagy into your life. There is no wrong goal. Autophagy can help you change your life and your health dramatically, including ways that you may not have been expecting.

Chapter 2: The Benefits of Autophagy

The benefits of autophagy are numerous enough that scientists are still engaged in elucidating them. To some, the benefits of this process are obvious as populations who live a life free from modern processed foods chocked full of chemicals and who are engaged in more physical activity than the average Westerner appear to be blessed with better health and longer lives than others. In this chapter, we will explore the major benefits of autophagy. The purpose of this discussion is not only to help you understand why you should consider ways that you can stimulate autophagy but also help you understand how much you have been missing by not thinking focusing on this important pathway.

You were introduced to the benefits of autophagy in the first chapter. These benefits include:

- Anti-aging capability
- Cancer-fighting ability
- Protection against neurodegenerative diseases, such as Parkinson's Disease
- Regulation of other cell organelles to enhance cellular function
- Protection against misfolded proteins that can cause amyloid diseases

- Improved neuroplasticity, brain function, and brain structure
- Strengthening of the immune system (directly and indirectly)
- Enhancement of the growth of heart cells
- Protecting DNA from degradation
- Protecting the body's organs and tissues from damage

These benefits will be explored in greater detail in this chapter; focusing on the major ways that autophagy can change lives.

Autophagy Can Help with Weight Loss (and Fat Loss)

Autophagy can lead to fat loss through its action in hepatic cells and other areas where fat is stored. The breakdown of fat is termed lipolysis, which literally means "breaking of fat (particles)." One of the remarkable aspects of autophagy is that it occurs in all cell types in the human body, so anywhere you have fat that is damaging to your body or unneeded autophagy can help you mobilize it. The best ways to achieve weight loss and fat loss with autophagy is through fasting, although exercise also works very well. This is why intermittent fasting combined with workout regimens like high-intensity interval training, or HIIT, has been found to lead to dramatic benefits in men and women regardless of the lifestyle of background.

Autophagy Can Improve Your Skin

Our skin is our largest organ. Many men and women do not think of their skin this way, but they should as it allows them to consider all the damage this organ takes from the sun, from chemicals, and from other factors in our environment. Autophagy is designed to help us undo some of the damage that we receive as a result of factors in our body as well as external factors like the sun. Harmful free radicals and other natural and unnatural elements in our environment need to be removed by the body, and autophagy is one of the major ways our body accomplishes this. Fasting, dieting, and exercise can give our skin a healthy glow and this is all thanks to autophagy.

Autophagy Can Improve Digestion

It is important for the cells of your digestive tract to be able to repair themselves and clear junk and other damaging particles. The cells of your mouth, esophagus, stomach, intestines, and other adjacent organs are all tasked with an important function, and that is to help your body process what it takes in and use those components for health. But in the process, your body exposes itself to things that can harm it. This makes autophagy particularly important in the GI tract as this organ (like the skin) is constantly being placed in harm's way. Finding ways to stimulate autophagy in your body can help you regulate your GI tract, leading to improved digestion and overall improved health.

Autophagy Can Improve Exercise Performance

Exercise performance tends to be improved when we engage in activities that activate our body's natural way of behaving. This is part of the reason why skipping breakfast before your morning workout, or even eating a light meal instead of gorging on fast food can make such a big difference. Our bodies are not expecting to be inundated with calories (especially not carbohydrates) early in the morning or before the activity so this tends to make us unregulated and less homeostatic because our body is forced to devote energy expenditure towards food breakdown instead of physical activity. Engaging in physical activity alone or combined with dieting and fasting stimulates autophagy and actually increases our exercise tolerance. This is partly due to more efficient use of energy.

Autophagy Can Prevent Cancer

Autophagy plays an essential role not only in removing damaging (or damaged) components from cells but in removing cells that are dysfunctional or should not be allowed to survive because they are not beneficial to the body. This is where the survival of the fittest analogy comes into play. Just as animals fight for survival in their environments, so too must cell fight for survival with the fewer fit cells being the ones to be removed.

Autophagy not only removes damaging components, but it removes cells that are not fit to stick around. It does this outside the specific programming of apoptosis, targeting cells that are normal enough but not quite fit. By doing this, autophagy can remove cells that have become cancerous or even before they reach this stage. This is part of the reason why cancer cells attempt to disrupt autophagy, a topic that will be discussed in greater detail later. By stimulating autophagy, you are not only strengthening your body's adaptive defenses, but you are helping to undo the deceptive tactics of cancer cells.

Autophagy Can Boost the Immune System

Autophagy has been shown to boost the actions of T1 and T2 helper cells. Autophagy has also been shown to stimulate other aspects of immune function and to play a role in the regulation of inflammation. Inflammation can occur as a result of trauma or injury, or it can be part of the immune system's response to infection. Stimulating autophagy can, therefore, protect you from infection as well as give you a healthier balance in times of inflammation. This means that inflammation can be localized to areas where it is needed, preventing you from feeling sicker than you need to be while your body is hard at work in clearing whatever ails it.

Autophagy Can Reduce the Risk of Neurodegenerative Diseases

Autophagy has neuroprotective effects, which means it can protect you from developing Parkinson's Disease, Alzheimer's

Disease, and other forms of dementia. This type of benefit is similar to some of the other benefits that have been mentioned on this list, as it is a function of the ability of this natural process to improve cellular function and longevity by helping it to remove poor components and recycle. Neurodegenerative diseases can be the result of a natural process of aging or they can be due to damage from free radicals, misfolded proteins, or other forms of stress. Just as you cannot prevent yourself from aging, you also cannot fully prevent yourself from being exposed to damaging particles. By stimulating autophagy, you are able to strengthen your body's natural way of protection, regardless of where your body's damage is coming from.

Autophagy Can Improve Your Metabolism

Autophagy is involved in lipolysis and other aspects of energy production. Indeed, autophagy is capable of using many of the components that it recycles for energy with the assistance of cell organelles, such as the lysosome, endoplasmic reticula, and lysosome. Stimulating autophagy is able to improve your metabolism by shifting your body in favor of recycling and energy production rather than energy storage in the form of fat cells or adipose tissue. Part of this picture also has to do with the ability of autophagy to improve insulin sensitivity.

Insulin insensitivity is the hallmark of type 2 diabetes, a condition characterized by continuously elevated levels of insulin in the bloodstream leading to the body developing resistance to insulin. High levels of insulin are in turn related to the body constantly being exposed to high levels of sugar in the blood. This means that stimulating autophagy by dieting and fasting is particularly beneficial, although exercise also can be useful here too. This improvement of metabolism – your body's breakdown of components as part of a healthy basal metabolic rate – has dramatic long term benefits regardless of what your goals are with autophagy.

Autophagy Can Improve Your Quality of Life

It has been demonstrated that stimulating autophagy can lead to men and women to feel subjectively healthier and more energetic. Part of this has to do with the ability of stimulation of this pathway to help with anxiety, depression, and other issues of mental health, but there are also aspects of autophagy that lead to wellbeing, a finding that is not entirely understood. Although science has identified dozens of autophagy genes, it is likely that the number of genes, proteins, and factors that play a role here will increase over time as this process because better understood. The improved sense of wellbeing, energy, and general health may be related to the CNS benefits that were discussed previously or they may be something different entirely. Studies suggest that how you stimulate autophagy is no important here, so exercise, fasting, dieting, or all three can be useful here.

Autophagy Can Lengthen Your Life

The anti-aging benefits of autophagy are a hotbed of research and discussion, and it is not difficult to understand why. Human beings have long searched for a miracle drug that can lengthen life and improve health, and it may turn out that that miracle drug is a process that our bodies have been engaging in since we were born. Autophagy is a natural way that our body protects us from damaging particles, infectious agents, and cancers. This process is also part of our normal process of recycling its components and using them to build other things and for energy.

As confusing as it may sound, autophagy has also been demonstrated to have anti-apoptotic effects. In other words, autophagy can extend life by discouraging apoptosis. By helping the body to achieve homeostasis and remove damaging particles, autophagy can prevent the activation of apoptosis triggers. Conversely, prolonged autophagy can actually stimulate apoptosis. The takeaway point here is that autophagy is designed to help us, and by stimulating it consistently and well we place ourselves on track for lives that are long, healthy, and filled with all of the other benefits of autophagy that were mentioned here.

Some of the benefits of autophagy actually involved multiple different specific benefits working together to create an overarching benefit, as is the case in anti-aging. As you have seen, autophagy actually causes anti-aging effects through several different mechanisms. Anti-aging can result from improved metabolism and cell turnover, or it can be a result of protection from neurodegenerative disease and cancer. Some aspects of anti-aging were not detailed here, including protection of DNA from damage. One way that autophagy protects DNA is through its protection from free radicals. These free radicals can shorten telomere and lead to DNA errors. Stimulating autophagy, therefore, can lead to greater telomere length, which indirectly increases longevity, a finding which some have informally labeled the telomere effect.

Other benefits of autophagy that have not been mentioned include the ability of this process to protect specific types of cells from damage or to improve them in dramatic ways, as is the case with the cells of the heart. The benefit of improvement in cardiovascular function through the action on heart cells is obvious, as the heart is an organ whose dysfunction is closely associated with morbidity. A particular area that will be touched on in this book is the ability of autophagy to aid men and women in achieving their specific health and fitness goals.

An understanding of what autophagy is and why it is beneficial is merely a precursor to a detailed explanation of why autophagy works. Most readers would not be motivated to dive into the gross details of autophagy without first getting a crash course on why autophagy is important. We have been exposed to the three main types of autophagy (macroautophagy, microautophagy, and chaperone-mediated autophagy) and a true understanding of this subject requires a more detailed examination of these subjects. In chapter three, you will gain more detail on the different types of autophagy and what they mean for you.

Chapter 3: How Autophagy Works

Autophagy exists because it works. Autophagy is a way that our body can repair damaged tissues or components without having to resort to apoptosis. Apoptosis should be thought of as a last resort. Programmed cell death is what our body must turn to when its components are absolutely beyond salvation. But sometimes cells and tissues are capable of being repaired and recycled. Indeed, sometimes the problem is an individual cell or an individual protein. If the body can merely get rid of this bad component then it cannot only restore its function, but it can improve it by removing a weak link in the chain. When we remember that these broken down components are then used to build new ones, the underlying benefits of this process to a complex organism like a human being becomes obvious.

In this chapter, we will examine how autophagy works by exploring the three major types of autophagy, namely macroautophagy, microautophagy, or chaperone-mediated autophagy (or CMA). These types of autophagy frequently work together to achieve the desired metabolic or exercise effect, but occasionally they have individual roles, as is the case of the role of microautophagy in helping the cardiovascular system deal with the drug rapamycin. Understanding the different types is the beginning of understanding in more detail the complexity of autophagy and how this complexity can really be distilled into three simple tools: fasting, dieting, and exercise.

The three main types of autophagy discussed here generally involve the operation of well-known cellular organelles, such as the lysosomes, endoplasmic reticulum, ribosomes, and mitochondria, although lesser-known structures such as the autophagosome and phagophore will also be discussed. As with other chapters in this book, some aspects of detailed terminology are explained in the glossary for reference purposes. The reason for exploring this subject is not to inundate the reader with details, but to help them make connections that may be of use to them later when it comes to being better understanding.

The Basics

Autophagy is a housekeeping tool that involves several organelles working together to accomplish the goal of keeping the cellular house in order. This may mean removing components that are damaging to the cell-like free radicals, processing degradation products so they can be reused for energy or repurposed, and even deciding that the cell itself should be degraded because it no longer meets the needs of the organism (in this case, the human body). The basic unit of autophagy function has been traditionally regarded as the lysosome, but further studies in recent decades have revealed that this organelle takes a back seat to a structure called the autophagosome.

This is not to say that the lysosome is not important. This organelle is extremely important, both in terms of the autophagy process and in related pathways like apoptosis. The lysosome is a double membrane structure that contains enzymes and other protein complexes that are capable of degradation and signaling. This allows the lysosome to work alone for breakdown, although it typically works in concert with other organelles. The name of the lysosome literally means "breaking (or breakdown) body."

The lysosome receives components for a breakdown from a double membrane vesicle known as the autophagosome. The presence of a double membrane is important as it allows components from outside the cell to be introduced into the interior of the cell, and it also allows the autophagosome to fuse with the lysosome, which contains enzymes and other necessary components. The movement of the autophagosome to the lysosome for breakdown and recycling occurs via the movement of microtubules which pull the organelles this way or that. This is the basic foundation for most autophagy pathways.

Macroautophagy

Macroautophagy is a process that utilizes several steps to trap components in the cytoplasm and recycle them. The first step is the formation of a structure called the isolation membrane. The formation of this structure is triggered by specific factors, some

42

of which will be discussed further shortly. This structure is formed within the cell's cytoplasm; that is, the "sea" of fluid within the cell, as opposed to extracellular fluid outside the cell membrane. Cells are very good at using membranes to separate extracellular components from intracellular ones. This is a means of regulating what is able to enter the cell and protecting the cell.

The second step after the formation of the isolation membrane is the formation of a structure known as the phagophore: a larger structure compared to the initial isolation membrane. The phagophore undergoes a process of expansion which leads to the engulfing of components in the cytoplasm and the formation of a third structure, the autophagosome. The autophagosome may be thought of as the basic essential structure of autophagy. This structure moves towards an important organelle called the lysosome, which results in the fusing of the autophagosome with the lysosome. The result is that the contents of the autophagosome are dumped into the lumen of the lysosome for degradation and recycling.

As it would be against the interests of our bodies to be degrading components willy nilly, macroautophagy is controlled in a highly nuanced manner by a series of triggers. Many of these triggers are in turn signaled and regulated by a number of proteins encoded in genes. Autophagy-related genes, or Atg, refer to proteins involved in the steps that lead to the formation of the autophagosome (via elongation).

Triggers of macroautophagy (in general terms) include:

- Fasting or starvation
- Lack of oxygen in the lungs
- Presence of reactive oxygen species
- Presence of infectious agents
- Therapeutic agents or drugs (like chemotherapy)

Microautophagy

In macroautophagy, the lysosome passively receives the vesicle (the autophagosome) containing the components intended for degradation and recycling. The autophagosome fuses with the lysosome in this case. In microautophagy, the lysosome is the main actor, directly engulfing the components in the cytosol that are intended for degradation. This process involves the double membrane of the lysosome folding in around the components that are being brought into the organelle, a process known as invagination. Like macroautophagy, this process is stimulated by specific triggers, of which factors in the environment are known to be significant.

Chaperone-mediated Autophagy (CMA)

Chaperone-mediated autophagy, or CMA, is an interesting pathway that is an active area of research. This type of autophagy also relies on the lysosome. In this pathway, particles designated for destruction are tagged with a molecule known as a chaperone. The chaperone is there to tag along, alerting the cell's organelles (particularly the lysosome), that this article is intended for destruction. The particle with the chaperone is recognized by receptors on the lysosomal membrane, which then invaginates the particle.

Other Types of Autophagy

There are several other types of autophagy that have been studied. Some of these fall under the three categories of macroautophagy, microautophagy, and chaperone-mediated autophagy, while others can be regarded as standalone pathways. For example, aggrephagy is regarded as a type of macroautophagy. Some lesser-known types of autophagy include.

Zymography: the detection and degradation of granules in the pancreas

Xenography: the degradation of toxic and infectious particles

Ribophagy: the breakdown of ribosomes

Pexography: the breakdown of peroxisomes (a type of organelle)

Mitophagy: the breakdown of mitochondria by lysosomes

Lipophagy: degradation of lipid droplets by autophagy

Chlorography: the protection from sunburn in some organisms

Aggrephagy: the degradation of cellular protein aggregates in macroautophagy

Autophagy Use in Therapeutic Agents

Autophagy has garnered attention in recent years for a number of reasons, not least of which is the potential use of autophagy as a target of therapeutic agents. That autophagy can be targeted for use by therapies for a wide number of purposes should come as a surprise to no one. Autophagy has already proven itself to be a tool that can be useful in cancer, weight loss, infection, and inflammation. In particular, autophagy has received attention for its potential uses in cancer.

Cancer therapies are often highly damaging to the person undergoing them. Chemotherapy and radiation can damage normal cells right alongside the abnormal ones, forcing scientists to find ways to streamline these sorts of therapies in order to spare normal tissue as much as possible. But therapies based on autophagy work by different means, and they have the potential of doing very little harm to non-cancerous cell. This is a function of autophagy's role as an entirely normal cellular process in human beings, which places this pathway in juxtaposition to chemotherapy and radiation which are essentially toxic therapies designed to be used against cancerous cells.

There are two main roles that therapeutic agents that operate based on autophagy can play in cancer. The first role is the use of therapeutic agents that attempt to stimulate autophagy and remove cancerous or otherwise dysfunction cells. In this scenario, a drug would stimulate autophagy in a particular cell type (like hepatic cells, for example), which would lead to the body naturally clearing cancerous cells and their components in the liver. The second role may be a little counterintuitive to some. This second role would involve therapeutic agents to block autophagy and trigger apoptosis in the cell.

Blocking autophagy may seem like something that you would not want to do, but in the case of cancer cells, there is a reason to take this route. Autophagy is also used to preserve cells that may be damaged or exposed to damaging particles, like infectious particles or free radicals. Autophagy does not only remove malfunctioning cells, but it saves those cells that can and should be salvaged. By inhibiting autophagy in cancer cells, the body will be able to trigger apoptosis in these cells and clear them, which would theoretically result in the clearing of a cancerous tumor. Indeed, cancer cells have evolved numerous ways of preserving themselves using genes and one of these ways is to prevent apoptosis from being triggered in cancerous cells.

Recall the apoptosis is programmed cell death, and it can be triggered by a number of factors and thresholds in the cell. Essentially, these triggers are designed to lead to cell death when it is clear that the cell has passed a threshold where it can (or should) be salvaged. The body is able to recognize that rapidly replicating or otherwise dysfunctional cells like cancerous tumors are "bad" and should be removed by the body using apoptosis. The cancer cells block apoptosis, causing these cells to be preserved when they should not be. By blocking autophagy in these cells, therapeutic agents can push the balance in favor of apoptosis.

Naturally, understanding autophagy deeply requires an in-depth understanding of how it can be stimulated or encouraged. Now that you understand the benefits of autophagy and the major pathways through which it operates you can begin to explore the major ways to stimulate this important process. In the next chapter, you will learn more about the three major mechanisms by which you can encourage autophagy in your body and reap all of the benefits.

Chapter 4: Stimulating Autophagy

When it comes to the benefits of autophagy, most people know about fasting. Indeed, fasting is so powerful a tool in humans that religious and spiritual groups the world over have incorporated fasting into their calendar of holy days and practices. But fasting is not the only way to stimulate autophagy. Indeed, specialists have come up with ways of mimicking fasting in order to trick the body into thinking it is fasting, allowing men and women who wish to benefit from fasting to partake of those benefits without having to deal with the downsides that usually come along with it.

Of course, most people choose to go about fasting the old fashion way; that is, to actually stop consuming calories. And the process of fasting is not as straightforward as some people like to think. For example, what should you drink when during a fast? Is it okay to consume decaffeinated products? What should you eat before you start fast? Your body's digestive process and other functions can be modified by fasting so what should you eat when breaking a fast? These questions and many others are perfectly legitimate ones, and they reveal that there is more to autophagy than most people think.

In fact, there is more to autophagy than you think. Autophagy is how your body incorporates Darwinian principles into its daily operations. In other words, autophagy is a type of survival of the fittest on a cellular level. Your body would not be a well-oiled machine if it was highly wasteful in its operations. For this reason, your body has learned to recycle components that it has consumed because it was weak, including not only components within the cell, but cells and tissues themselves.

The purpose of this is to make the body better. It is a selfish process that allows cells to survive because they are more suited to the purposes that the body needs them for. This allows the body itself to be better at surviving compared to other "bodies" (which is why the process involved in the first place). This is all part of a larger homeostatic process. The human body is constantly engaged in a balancing game of breaking things down and building them up. This breaking down and the building is balanced in order to achieve the homeostasis the body needs to survive as long as it can.

A good example of this is the bone. The bone has cells in its marrow called osteoblasts and osteoclasts. Osteoblasts are the cells responsible for laying new bone, while osteoclasts are the cells responsible for breaking down bone. Now it may seem as if breaking down bone may be a bad thing. It is if this breaking down is not balanced with building up bone, as is the case in osteoporosis. The reverse situation is also true. Building up too much bone can be bad as it can lead to bones that abnormally think and less functional than our body needs to be.

The normal situation (and the desired one) is for the body to be constantly breaking down and building up the bone to a certain degree in order to maintain bone homeostasis. This equilibrium allows the bone to be remodeled in response to stress. So if you ride horses a lot, the osteoclasts break down your bone while the osteoblasts reform bone that will take a slightly different shape in response to the stress of the horse's back against the long bones of your legs. The result is the bow-leggedness that we associate with cowboys and other prolonged riders of horses.

Stimulating autophagy is therefore about tapping into this type of homeostasis. It is not an all or nothing equation, which is typical for the human body (i.e. non-all-or-nothing situations). Life on Earth is about balance and even life in your body is about a measure of balance. Your goal, therefore, is to tap into this balance and shift the scale in favor of those things that encourage the sorts of things that you want. Let us jog our memories and recall what some of the reasons for wanting to stimulate autophagy are. The reasons why you want to activate or stimulate autophagy include:

- Greater weight loss or fat loss
- Improved metabolism and insulin sensitivity
- Improved immune functioning
- Improved DNA repair and stabilization
- Anti-aging effects
- Anti-cancer effects

- Improved exercise tolerance
- Improved cardiovascular function
- Improved nervous system functioning
- Protection from neurodegenerative disease
- Protection from infection
- Improved sense of health and wellness
- Improved quality of life

These are the sorts of things that most men and women would want. There are few people living today who would admit to wanting a short life filled with cardiovascular disease, neurodegenerative disease, poor DNA stability, and insulin resistance. Regardless of what your specific goals are, there is certainly a role played by autophagy as a constantly occurring process in the achievement of your goals. In this chapter, we will review the three main ways that you can stimulate autophagy in order to improve your goals.

But before we do that, let us spend a moment thinking about what stimulating or activating autophagy means. All it really refers to is shifting the equilibrium balance in favor of autophagy as opposed to maintenance of poor cellular and tissue function and eventually apoptosis. Recall that apoptosis is programmed cell death, and this happens when your body is not able to salvage a cell because it is old, poorly functioning or damaged. Your goal is to encourage autophagy rather than apoptosis because the former is associated with improved health outcomes and longevity while the latter is not.

It is also important to remember that autophagy is stimulated by general environmental or contextual factors, specific environmental changes, and specific enzymes and proteins related to the first two states. So starvation and fasting are general environmental (for the body) factors that encourage autophagy while drinking green tea gives you specific chemicals that also stimulate autophagy without actually causing an "environmental" factor change in the body. Many of these triggers of autophagy involved an important protein called AMP-activated kinase, which is responsible for stimulating autophagy on a molecular level.

So what are the major ways of stimulating autophagy? These should not come as a complete surprise. They are listed below:

- Fasting
- Dieting
- Exercise

Under the scope of dieting, we include intermittent fasting and extended water fasting, which will be covered in more detail in this book. Under the heading of dieting, we include eating regimens like the well-known Ketogenic diet, which involves consuming a diet very low in carbohydrates or no carbs at all. Related diets include the Atkins diet and the Paleo diet. Exercise is a means of stimulating autophagy that is often ignored, though, as we have seen it is an important trigger because of its ability to improve metabolism and other processes closely tied to autophagy.

Fasting

Fasting is regarded as the best way to stimulate autophagy. Although different studies have different recommendations regarding how long you can fast, some in the industry argue that a single 18-hour fast can be enough to kill cancer cells in the body. Others have recommended longer periods of fasting, such as a day-long fast, with days of more regular eating before and after. It is interesting to ponder whether the incorporation of fasting rites into religious practices actually represents a way that early modern humans managed to incorporate their observations about health and longevity into their religious practices and taboos.

Fasting essentially is a period in which you deprive your body of calories of any kind. Fasting stimulates the release of factors that activate autophagy, like AMP-activated kinase. These periods of fasting have numerous benefits aside from just losing weight, although even this is mediated by autophagy which is involved in the process of lipolysis (the breakdown of fat or adipose tissue). Many men and women fear to fast because of misconceptions they have about it. Fasting does not have to be for a prolonged period. Indeed, the most popular type of fasting in the health and fitness community is intermittent fasting, which involves incorporating hours without eating into your daily eating schedule (which will be discussed in more detail later).

Dieting

Dieting is also able to stimulate autophagy by similar means to fasting. Although fasting is regarded as the gold standard when it comes to stimulation of this important pathway, many men and women are able to achieve very dramatic results with dieting because it also taps into the same metabolic and tissue breakdown pathways as fasting (although in a less dramatic fashion).

This is an opportune time to talk about the Ketogenic diet, which will be discussed at length in a later chapter. The Ketogenic diet is designed to place the body in ketosis, which involves the release of molecules called ketone bodies from the liver. Ketosis has been associated with a wide variety of health benefits, almost as many as autophagy. The big problem with ketosis is that prolonged ketosis can be damaging to the body, and some medical conditions render ketosis life-threatening because of morbidity concerns (as in type 2 diabetes).

There is a lot of misinformation out there about the Ketogenic diet. The Ketogenic diet has become very popular very quickly because of the dramatic effect it can have on changing your body. Many men and women have gone from obesity to a normal BMI with Keto. The benefits of the Ketogenic diet include:

- Reduction in blood glucose
- Increase in insulin sensitivity (and reduced insulin levels)
- Improved organ functioning
- Improved concentration
- Lower triglyceride levels
- Lower blood pressure
- Lower blood sugar

Exercise

Exercise is a stimulator of autophagy that is easy to overlook. Many people attempt dieting and exercise and do not lose weight (a common goal), which is why they often look askance at programs that focus on these two things. But an exercise regimen that is consistent and involves a measure of muscle strain and cardiovascular activity can dramatically benefit the body in ways outside of the desired weight loss or muscle building. Indeed, many people fall prey to adopting a workout program that does not place enough emphasis on intensity. Your goal in your exercise program should be to get your heart rate up. It is this stress on the body that leads the body to change itself in ways that benefit you.

Much attention has been paid lately to HIIT, or high-intensity interval training. A program of HIIT cannot only dramatically change your body's appearance but increase aerobic and anaerobic capacity. That is, the ability to tolerate exercise in cases where your muscles have adequate oxygen, and in cases where they do not. HIIT and other types of exercise increase the rate of autophagy, which improves exercise tolerance, improves concentration, and increases the rate of fat breakdown (or lipolysis).

A question that is important to ask is how much HIIT is too much. It is important to remember that HIIT is meant to be done in intervals, which means that not all of your workouts (or sets within a workout) or at the same high level of intensity. Not only does prolonged high intensity weaken your muscles and increase the risk of injury, but prolonged high intensity can actually lead to apoptosis, which is certainly something that you want. You can think of this as another case where equilibrium or homeostasis is coming into play.

Muscle growth is the result of muscle breakdown which forces the muscle to grow. In other words, when you are working out intensely, you are stressing and breaking down muscle fibers, which force them to become hypertrophied so that they can better handle stress in the future. You want to shift the balance in favor of slightly increased breakdown so that during periods of rest you can have greater repair. This is an example of using your body's normal equilibrium in the right way. But if you were to be too intense in your training, you would be causing an overwhelming shift towards breakdown, not allowing your body to recover, which leads to permanent injuries (like muscle tears) and apoptosis.

Studies of moderate exercise and high-intensity interval training have shown differences that are based on autophagy. Both exercise programs cause an improvement in immune functioning, and of course can cause things like weight loss and improved body image, but there are powerful results specifically associated with HIIT. These results are consistent with what we would expect from an exercise program that is specifically using autophagy to impact the body during exercise. These benefits include:

- Better aerobic metabolism
- Better aerobic performance
- Better pulmonary ventilation
- Better peak VO2 (volume of oxygen)

Chapter 5: Water Fasting and Ketosis Diets

One of the advantages of autophagy as a solution to your health problems or goals is that it can be stimulated in various ways, as we have seen. We have discussed fasting at length as a trigger for autophagy in the human body, and we will discuss exercise (in addition to intermittent fasting) in the next chapter. The purpose of this chapter is to explore some of the major ways that dieting can be used to stimulate autophagy: one of the body's major pathways that can lead to targeted fat loss.

There is a thin line between a fast and a diet. Most fasts discussed in this book are really diets that involve periods of fasting. This is particularly true of intermittent fasting, which has become one of the most popular ways to lose fat and preserve muscle in the health and fitness community. If you are thinking that dieting versus fasting is really a matter of semantics than you are right. Most fasting is really dieting because if you were to fast forever than that would actually be starvation. Most people who "fast" on purpose intend to break that fast, which means they have to put some thought into such things as what to eat before the fast and how to break the fast (i.e. what to eat afterward). In this chapter, we focus on dieting, specifically two diets whose effects are closely linked to autophagy: extended water fasting and ketosis diets.

Ketosis diets are really an umbrella term for diets that seek to achieve just that: ketosis. Ketosis is the state of ketone body production in your bodies. Ketone bodies are normally produced from fat mobilized in the liver in response to starvation. Ketosis can sometimes be a bad thing, as is the case with type I diabetics who present to the emergency room in Ketogenic shock. But ketosis is also associated with positive states in the body, which has led to ketosis being used for weight loss and a host of other health benefits. In this chapter, we deal specifically with the Ketogenic diet, although other diets like the Atkins Diet also operate via ketosis.

Extended Water Fasting

Water fasting uses nutrient deprivation to trigger autophagy in the body. Water is an essential element for human survival, but it does not contain any calories and cannot be used for energy. This means that you can drink as much water as you want and still be in starvation as far as the body is concerned because you have not taken in any products that can be used for energy. Ultimately, this is what the body uses "food" for: as a source of energy and other essential nutrients and building blocks the body requires.

A water fasting diet is, therefore, a diet that involves supplanting meals with water in order to maintain the body in a fast for a prolonged period. In this regard, a water fasting diet is not too different from an intermittent fasting diet, which will be discussed shortly (in the next chapter). Intermittent fasting involves separating periods of eating by periods of fasting, which can take up a whole day or just part of a day. This can also be done on a water fasting diet.

Your water fasting diet can take up a portion of your day or it can last for 1-2 days. A longer fast with water is known as an extended water fasting diet, and some people choose to fast this way for 7 days or longer. Seven days is a big number as studies have shown that this number of days is enough to completely remove cancerous cells from your body (if you are in a precancerous state). This is because cancer cells are rapidly dividing and cannot survive without nutrients over this period of time.

Your water fasting can take any form that you would like it to. Naturally, you will have to make sure that you are drinking adequate quantities of water or you will really find yourself in trouble. Diets like this work because during this period of fast your body is using autophagy for lipolysis and other metabolic processes that lead to weight loss. Some people feel that water helps them to feel full, which is why water diets can be effective rather than a dry fast. Choose the duration of water fasting that works for you, making sure to be start off slow and be realistic with your expectations or risk backsliding into your poor eating habits.

The Ketogenic Diet

The Ketogenic diet is probably the best known of several diets that operate by triggering ketosis. Ketosis is a period of altered body functioning that is triggered by the presence of ketone bodies in the bloodstream. Indeed, ketosis merely means the state of having ketones in the blood. There are three ketone bodies whose production is triggered by prolonged periods of starvation or fasting. The three ketone bodies produced during ketogenesis are acetoacetate, beta-hydroxybutyrate, and acetone. Although prolonged ketosis can be harmful and even fatal, there are positive benefits that are seen in ketosis. Some of these overlap with the benefits of intermittent fasting and autophagy in general.

Ketosis is triggered by a state of extremely low carbohydrates. For this reason, the Ketogenic diet and other diets that operate based on ketosis like Atkins have their clients consume diets extremely low in carbohydrates. Carbs are considered bad because they increase your circulating glucose concentration and cause major problems with insulin sensitivity and metabolism. At the practical level, the body stores excess sugar as fat, which is not what are most people going on a diet want?

In the Ketogenic diet, an eating program high in fat and protein is consumed. Fat and protein do not cause problems with metabolism and insulin so they are not problematic in this protocol. Also, the idea is to replace carbs with other sources of calories, and these are the two other macronutrients that the body can resort to for energy. Ketogenic diets are very low in carbohydrates. Less than 10% of total daily calories are consumed from carbohydrates. So if your caloric intake should be 2000 calories for the day, this means that you would only be consuming 200 calories from carbohydrates, which is about 50 grams. That is less than one 16 oz. bottle of soda. Most people on Keto consume even fewer carbs, i.e. 100 calories or 25 grams of carbohydrates.

It is important to be realistic when starting any diet. This means determining that a diet fits in with any health problems you have. But it also means thinking about whether you will be able to stick to the diet and perhaps what things you need to do before starting the diet. Keto is not for everyone, but those who have tried it and reaped the benefits swear by it.

Chapter 6: Autophagy for Muscle Mass

Autophagy is just as useful for preserving muscle as it is at for losing weight. This is part of what makes autophagy-dependent programs a lifestyle rather than merely a diet. In stimulating autophagy through fasting, dieting, or exercise you create a new paradigm for your body that triggers a series of changes that leads to an entirely new health outlook. Men and women who experience fatigue, a weakened immune system, and obesity can suddenly find that they are losing weight, more energetic, and less prone to colds than they had formerly been. And all of this is due to finding ways of incorporating autophagy stimulation into their lives.

As you have already seen, activating autophagy is as simple as remembering three simple words: dieting, fasting, and exercise. We can also add a fourth word – food – but technically this is part of dieting. Food will be explored further in the next chapter as it is a simple and reliable way to stimulate autophagy. Dieting and food also allow you to improve your metabolism, which will not only lead you to look better and feel better but to have more energy and longevity. Some even describe a glow that people have because of autophagy. This is not pseudoscience. Autophagy has been shown to provide benefits to skin, hair, and other organs: all as a result of the improved functioning of the body that results from careful and considerate stimulation of this process.

Some of you may be wondering what autophagy can possibly have to do with working out and muscle mass. It has everything to do with it, to be honest. Autophagy improves your metabolism, increases your insulin sensitivity, and burns fat through direct lipolysis. These are all things that men and women interested in building muscle, or merely in looking better and losing weight, hope to achieve. Stimulation of autophagy pathways is essential to anyone looking to improve their bodies by adding muscle without having to resort to illicit performance-enhancing drugs.

Intermittent Fasting

This is a convenient juncture to begin the discussion of intermittent fasting, one of the most popular diets in the health and fitness industry right now. Indeed, intermittent fasting is popular even outside the fitness industry as many men and women have discovered how this diet can dramatically alter their bodies and their lives. Intermittent fasting has the term fasting in it, but it really out to be thought of as a type of diet. This is because, in intermittent fasting, one of the most important things that the dieter needs to do is to learn to pay attention to macronutrients as well as total caloric intake.

Indeed, it is a myth in both the Ketogenic diet and intermittent fasting that the total amount of calories consumed is unimportant. Although some people who consume high caloric diets as part of their sport – like professional athletes, bodybuilders, and powerlifters – might pay less attention their calories than others would this does not mean they are unimportant. In intermittent fasting, it is important to pay attention to the total number of calories consumed in a day and when you are consuming them as part of keeping track of your macronutrients (or macros) and in order to make sure that you are eating enough in order to meet your respective macro needs for the day.

In other words, in intermittent fasting, you have to pay attention to calories or risk finding yourself hungry because you did not properly estimate how much you need to eat during your eating window. This brings us to a discussion of what precisely intermittent fasting is and how it works. Intermittent fasting is essentially what it sounds like. It is a diet (or eating program) that involves a period of fasting separated by periods of eating. The duration of the fasting period can vary based on the specific regimen adopted by the dieter. Intermittent fasting is usually divided into two types:

- Alternate-day fasting
- Time-restricted eating

These are similar. They only differ in terms of whether the fasting lasts for an entire day or part of the day. In alternate-day fasting, the dieter spends an entire day (24 hours) without eating, while in time-restricted feeding the day is divided into periods of eating and fasting. Both alternate-day fasting and time-restricted feeding are popular ways of going about this diet with men and women finding ways of making the eating schedule work in their often hectic lives.

Time-restricted feeding, however, has received more attention from the health and fitness media because it has attracted a number of influential supporters in the community. This type of diet is popular for bodybuilders and fitness competitors who are looking to shed fat and preserve as much muscle as possible. Although calories are important and need to be planned carefully, this type of diet can allow you to consume high calories as long as they are within a certain window.

So how does the time-restricted feeding type of intermittent fasting diet work? It is pretty simple. The dieter comes up with a particular window in hours that they will be allowed to eat in the day and fasts for the rest of the day. A popular type is the so-called 16/8 split. This protocol involves consuming all of your meals in an 8-hour window and fasting for the remaining 16 hours. This would take the form of eating, say, between 11AM and 7PM (an 8-hour window) and fasting the rest of the day. This split has been shown to be very effective at shedding fat, but you can use whatever window you choose. It can be a 20/4 window, in which you only eat for four hours in the day, or it can be more or less restrictive.

Intermittent fasting brings with it all of the benefits of autophagy that have been discussed in other areas of this book. It also has some benefits of its own. These have been elucidated by vigorous study both inside the fitness community and outside of it. The benefits of intermittent fasting are numerous. Here are some of them:

- Improved fat loss
- Improved cardiovascular functioning
- Improved glucose control
- Increased lifespan
- Reduced muscle loss
- Reduced hunger
- Improved metabolism
- Improved self-image and energy
- Reduced risk of cancer
- Reduced risk of neurodegenerative disease

Incorporating Intermittent Fasting into Your Workout Plan

If you have an active workout regimen (or an active life), it is important to choose a diet that works with your workout and other responsibilities. Fasting is difficult for many people because they feel they need the calories that come from food for their occupation, their workout regimen, or just for the energy to get them through a day filled with screaming children or obnoxious bosses and coworkers. There is nothing wrong with that. Intermittent fasting can allow you to have shorter periods of "fasting" in your day so you are able to eat as you need.

The key is to come up with a schedule that fits with your life. For example, if you need to be at work at 8AM and you typically go to the gym at 6AM, perhaps you should consider a 16/8 intermittent fasting split with an eating window between 7:30AM and 3:30PM. This will allow you to squeeze your eating period into your busy day. For those whose obligations are later in the day, you may want to push your eating window back a little so that you are not engaging in heavy activities on an empty stomach.

Little side notes about eating before a workout: many fitness enthusiasts have found advantages to working out on an empty stomach. Although your energy levels may be slightly reduced at first because you are used to having sugar constantly in your bloodstream, it has been shown that working out on an empty stomach increases your metabolism, improves insulin sensitivity, and provides a host of other benefits. Consider working out on an empty stomach if you work out first thing in the morning. You could always have your first meal in your window after your workout.

Other things to keep in mind here will be touched on in the Frequently Asked Questions section. Some are curious about what they should eat before a fast, after a fast, or whether it is safe for them to fast. These questions and many more will be answered. All you have to do is keep reading.

Chapter 7: Foods that Stimulate Autophagy

Most of you reading this book are likely doing so not because you plan on writing a paper and submitting it to a journal. Most likely you have a specific goal that you plan to achieve with Autophagy and you are looking for tools to help you achieve that goal. Your goal may be weight loss, it may reduction in cancer risk, or it may just be feeling better through dieting or fasting. If any of these are your goals, thinking about the sorts of food you should eat is clearly something that would be beneficial to you.

In this chapter, we will review some of the major foods that have been shown to stimulate autophagy. We will choose several foods to explore in detail. Naturally, all of the foods that play a role in stimulating autophagy cannot be examined in detail because if they were, you would find yourself reading a book solely about that. So what are the foods that you can incorporate into your diet in order to stimulate autophagy? Some of the major foods in this category include:

- Ginger
- Green tea
- Reishi mushrooms
- Turmeric/curcumin

These foods each stimulate autophagy although they do it in different ways. Some readers may notice that several foods on this list are regarded as superfoods that provide a wide host of benefits. These are foods that are consumed in some traditional cuisines, especially in East Asia and South Asia. These are areas where residents most likely identified early on that these superfoods provided benefits for health and longevity, even if they may not have understood why exactly in these early days.

You may be asking yourself how you can incorporate these foods into your diets. Some of these, like green tea, are easily incorporated. Drinking one to two glasses of green tea in the first half of your day is not difficult to do. It might be a better idea to drink tea in the first portion of your day because the caffeine in your tea can keep you up at night. There are also are some particular aspects of green tea to keep in mind (which will be explored shortly). Ginger and Reishi mushrooms are ingredients that can be conveniently added to a wide variety of dishes, such as salads or soups. Turmeric/curcumin is a dry spice that also can be added to meat dishes or a wide variety of other dishes. Getting a benefit from these does not require that you go overboard, although if you find that you like one or more of these and would like to add more to your mealtimes, it is generally safe to do this in the case of the four foods provided here.

Ginger

Ginger is one of those foods that are so good for you that it is difficult to overstate its power. Indeed, ginger has been shown to have dramatic anti-oxidant benefits that place it as a great resource for those dealing with an infection. Ginger has also been purported to increase longevity. This last claim should come as no surprise as research has shown that ginger directly stimulates autophagy, which will be explained further shortly. Ginger exists in the form of a thick and fragrant root. It has a characteristic odor and taste. Ginger together with honey is a traditional and very effective remedy for resolving the common cold.

For our purposes, it is important to note that ginger contains a number of important compounds. These include gingerol as well as a group of compounds known as shogaols. 6-shogoal is the most common of this group of chemicals. These chemicals are similar in structure to gingerol. 6-shogaol is believed to be the more important compound in autophagy. It has been shown to induce autophagy in cancer cells, but not programmed cell death (apoptosis). This has been shown to be particularly powerful in lung cancers. Incorporating ginger in your diet will help you boost your immune system and fight off cancer, all through the power of autophagy.

Green Tea

Many volumes have been written about tea and its benefit. Here, we focus on one of these teas: green tea. Green tea is a popular variety although it does compete for sales with some of the other varieties. Indeed green tea is just one of many different commercially available teas that have been demonstrated to provide health benefits to those who drink it. Green tea also has antioxidant properties and is believed to have anti-aging benefits. It boosts autophagy in the skin and can improve organ function, too. In fact, one should keep in mind that even if particular foods are associated with particular benefits, because they stimulate autophagy they are likely to provide some of the other autophagy benefits too (like improved metabolism) even if it is to a slightly lesser degree.

The compound that we are interested in is called EGCG. Epigallocatechin gallate, or EGCG, is a catechin found in teas. EGCG has a polyphenol structure and it is the most abundant catechin found in tea. Also contained in other foods, EGCG has been studied extensively because of its many potential health benefits. EGCG stimulates autophagy in hepatic cells leading to lipolysis, or lipid breakdown. EGCG accomplishes this by increasing the concentration of AMP-activated protein kinase. As we have seen, AMPK is a direct stimulator of autophagy

Reishi Mushrooms

Mushrooms can easily be added to many different meals. Reishi mushrooms would break a fast although it is worth it because of its autophagy benefits. Adding Reishi mushrooms to your diet has been shown to reduce the incidence of colon cancer. Reishi mushrooms do not demonstrate their effects through AMP Kinase, but through another pathway called the mitogen pathway. Reishi mushrooms have also been shown to have a role in stabilizing the nervous system. Adding this mushroom to your diet really can go a long way in helping you feel better and experience positive health outcomes.

Turmeric/curcumin

Turmeric/curcumin is a spice that is commonly found in South Asian cuisine. Indeed, in some parts of India turmeric is put in most dishes. Curcumin in turmeric does not have the best bioavailability, but this can be increased by consuming black pepper along with this orange/brown spice. Turmeric is a component of Indian Ayurvedic Medicine as are the other items in this list of autophagy stimulators. Turmeric specifically is regarded as having great neuroprotective effects and anti-inflammatory powers. Turmeric also plays an anti-cancer role through the mediation of AMPK (activating it through phosphorylation). Adding turmeric to your intermittent fasting or Ketogenic diet dishes can go a long way in further boosting the autophagy benefits you already expect.

Chapter 8: Stimulating Autophagy by Mimicking Fasting

Imitating fasting with the so-called Fasting Mimicking Diet is an option for men and women who would like the benefits of fasting, but may have reasons why fasting is not the best choice for them. Fasting is regarded as the gold standard in terms of stimulating autophagy because of its demonstrated use in triggering the body to remove damaged, poorly functioning, or dysfunctional components, such as cancer cells. But autophagy can also be stimulated well by diet and exercise, and in the case of the Fasting Mimicking Diet, the goal is to create a diet that resembles fasting without actually being fasting.

Recall that the idea behind fasting is that it replicates how our human ancestors would have eaten tens of thousands of years ago. At this time, human beings would have lived primarily as hunter-gatherers and not in the settled agricultural societies that characterize the way nearly all humans on Earth live today. This means that humans would not have had access to storehouses filled with grain, sugar cane, processed foods, and all the other goodies that many people take for granted today. If you wanted to eat, you would have had to hunt or fish your quarry or risk starvation.

Now, this type of life may seem harsh, but our bodies adapted to survive in this type of environmental context. It is not too different from how apex predators like lions and tigers live in their environments today. They spend much of their day sleeping or guarding their territory (essentially a fasting period), while they devote a portion of their day to hunting and eating. Naturally, when a lion hunts he's or she is generally obeying both a predatory urge and a physical urge. He or she is hungry. This means that the fasting period actually serves to motivate the lion to hunt and hunt well. You rarely see obese or out of shape lions because their way of life demands that they are a well-oiled machine.

Well, human beings were once not too different from these apex predators. We also used to spend much of our days sleeping or guarding are territories, and we would have hunted on an empty stomach. Obesity would have been rare in social groups where food was not instantly available and men and women would have had to hunt for survival. Today, we are constantly exposed to food in frankly enormous quantities, including high concentrations of sugar that would have baffled our ancestor. What some diets do is focus on what we take into our body as a way of preventing the lowered metabolism and energy drain that comes from eating diets high in carbohydrates.

The Fasting Mimicking Diet allows men and women who are interested in reaping the benefits of diets like the Ketogenic diet or intermittent fasting to tap into those benefits without all of the restrictions. The Fasting Mimicking Diet involves devoting five days out of a 30-day period to caloric restriction similar to what is seen in Keto while the remaining 25 days are less restrictive. The idea here is to place the body in something akin to ketosis in order to mobilize adipose (fat) stores for energy rather than the circulating blood sugars that most people who eat sugar and carbs constantly use for energy. This excess sugar is not only used for energy but stored as fat which is counterproductive and leads to obesity. By cutting out sugar sources, you force your body to look to other more natural energy sources. This leads to benefits like fat mobilization (lipolysis) through autophagy as well as other benefits like improved insulin sensitivity.

Basics of the Fasting Mimicking Diet

The essential fact to remember about the Fasting Mimicking Diet is that during your five days of the fasting mimicking you are drastically reducing your caloric intake but not actually going on a fast. A fast means that you are not taking in any calories at all, and during your fasting-mimicking days, you would be taking in perhaps as little as 500 calories. Five hundred calories would be equivalent to one large cheeseburger at a fast-food restaurant or a large highly processed pastry (that is high in fat and carbohydrates).

As the Ketogenic diet, what you eat during your fasting-mimicking days is important as the idea is to trick your body into thinking that you are fasting. You do this by eating a diet that is relatively low in carbohydrates, but not as low as it would be in Keto. Recall that the hallmark of Keto is that carb intake is reduced to almost zero. In Fasting Mimicking, you may take in about 30% of your calories from carbohydrates. It is okay to do this because your total caloric intake is so low (between 500 to 1000 calories for five days).

The idea here is that this period of low calories is recognized by the body as starvation, which is the essential goal of a fast. Fasting and starvation are distinguished by the body merely by duration. For example, any period of no food is technical "starvation" to the body although we tend to use this term only to refer to periods where individuals have no caloric intake for a prolonged period usually due to circumstances outside of their control. Prolonged starvation can lead to syndromes like kwashiorkor or marasmus that are seen in countries experiencing drought or other calamities.

To return to our main point: tricking your body into thinking that it is in starvation because of days of low calories triggers autophagy. Most people on the Fasting Mimicking Diet do it because they want to lose weight, but all of the other benefits of autophagy can be reaped here, too. This is a recurring theme in this book. Autophagy confers a host of benefits to the person who stimulates it, and you might find that you reap positive health advantages that you had not anticipated, like a sense of energy and well-being.

The main benefit of the Fasting Mimicking Diet is that you can enter something like a fast without some of the downsides of a fast (or starvation). Some people may find fasting difficult because they have never done it before. Others may have health concerns that render fasting inadvisable. The Fasting Mimicking Diet allows you to stimulate autophagy similar to how you would in a fast. Again, research suggests that fasting of 18 to 24 hours is the best way to stimulate autophagy (and reap its benefits), but not everyone can do this. Some people use the Fasting Mimicking Diet as a starting point to attempting fasting in the future.

Example of a Fasting Mimicking Diet Protocol

A typical Fasting Mimicking Diet protocol consists of 5 consecutive days of fasting-mimicking followed by 25 days without fasting mimicking. Most practitioners of this diet carefully follow their macronutrients (macros) just as they would in the Ketogenic diet. Typically the first of the five days is lower on carbohydrates, but the carbs are increased slightly in the following days. There are different ways to go about this diet, but an example of a diet using this protocol is shown below. The percentage shown is the relative percentage of total calories for the day from that macronutrient. Recall that the three main macronutrients are fat, protein, and carbohydrates.

First Day (Day 1):

A total of five to six calories total for each pound of body weight, so about 800 calories for a 160-pound person

Fat: 60%

Protein: 10%

Carbohydrate: 30%

Following Days (Days 2 through 5):

A total of three to four calories in total for each pound of body weight, so about 480 calories for a 160-pound person

Fat: 50%

Protein: 10%

Carbohydrate: 40%

Chapter 9: Tips to Help with Fasting

Some people learn best with tips. Let's face it, there is a lot to learn about autophagy, and no one is expected to be an expert after reading about the subject for an hour or two. You will learn the most about this process after you have given stimulating it a try. Tips can help you whether your goal is to lose weight or too fast for days and days in order to kill cancer cells in your body. Here are some tips to help get you started.

Tip 1. You do not have to skip meals in order to fast.

Although fasting means that you are not eating, it does not necessarily mean that you have to skip a meal. What are we talking about here? People who intermittent fast and have a 16/8 split, for example, are still able to eat a normal (or relatively normal) three meals a day. They just have to do this in a smaller window than they normally might. So your breakfast might be at 10 AM, your lunch might be at 1:30, and your dinner might be at 5:30. Fasting is a different word from "starvation" for a reason. Fasting does not have to mean that you are miserable.

Tip 2. Having coffee before you start your fast (or something else with fat in it) can keep you satiated.

There is a lot of talk about whether or not coffee drinking should be considered breaking a fast. Part of this subject will be discussed in more detail shortly. In truth, there are some calories in coffee, but they are so low (generally less than 100 calories) that they are not counted by many people who fast. But for the purpose of this trip, we are thinking about ways that you can work coffee in before you fast. If you have coffee right before a fast it can help keep you satiated, especially if it contains some cream or other additives with a little added fat in it.

Tip 3. Drinking water during your fast can help you feel fuller.

Water fasting is a thing for a reason. No, not because some people are lunatics who like to drink water until it makes them sick (which is actually a thing). Water can help you feel fuller. There is some debate as to whether this is due to receptors in your stomach being stretched by the volume of water or because of some other reason, but all you need to know is that works. It may not be a good idea to replace all of your next five meals with water when you are just starting out with this, but it is something to keep in mind. Having a tall glass of water can help you stave off your hunger when your goal is to fast for a short while longer.

Tip 4. Work your way up to longer fasts rather than jumping into a long fast early on.

Taking baby steps is always a good idea. When it comes to fasting, this means not jumping into a highly restrictive fast, but working your way up to it. It is not difficult to do. Indeed, some people do this by first engaging in an autophagy diet like intermittent fasting and then working their way up to a whole day fast or longer. Again, you always have the option of drinking water as part of your fast thereby incorporating a water fasting diet. Most people who fast for days and days started out where you might be now - a little overweight and wondering if it is possible to make a major change in their life. The answer is "yes," it is possible.

Tip 5. Eating a pinch of salt during a fast can quench your hunger pangs.

Some fasting experts recommend eating a pinch of salt during periods when you are tempted to break your fast. Salt is sodium chloride, which means it contains two ions that are essential in your body's homeostasis. Sodium chloride not only can satiate your taste buds, but it can help you feel fuller (and better) by keeping the water in your body. Have you noticed that when you drink large quantities of water you tend to urinate it out relatively quickly? That is because your body needs sodium chloride in order to keep the water in your body's cells and tissues. So here is a little trick. If you are having problems with your fast, try adding a pinch of salt.

Tip 6. Apple cider vinegar may break your fast but it will help you while intermittent fasting.

Apple cider vinegar contains acetic acid which assists in vitamin and mineral uptake in the body. The acetic acid in the vinegar will help your body to absorb the vitamins and minerals that your body consumed in foods hours earlier. Apple cider vinegar also contains polyphenols that boost the immune system. Besides that, some people like the taste of apple cider vinegar so consuming this can help you get the most out of what you have eaten earlier so you will not feel as hungry.

It is a matter of debate whether or not apple cider vinegar will break a fast. Some in the health industry argue that it does not contain enough calories to impact insulin so it will not break a fast. Others say that apple cider vinegar is not zero calories, and even one calorie is enough to break a fast. Even if you drink this right before you start a fast you can have a benefit during your fast. To incorporate this type of vinegar into your fasting regimen. You will not regret it.

Tip 7. Adding a pinch of sea salt to your water can help you maintain your fast.

Salt does not have to be a bad thing. We have already spoken about adding a pinch of salt, but it is important here to talk about the benefits of all-natural options during your fast. Processed products, like artificial sweeteners, can actually cause problems with your fast because they can derail your metabolism. Even salt can have other things added to it that make it more than just regular salt. So if you are planning to use salt to help you along in your fast, try sea salt or another of nature's varieties of this substance.

Tip 8. Avoid supplements like branched-chain amino acids during your fast because these will cause an insulin spike.

Whether or not to take supplements is always a big question when it comes to fast. Many people continue to take supplements during their fast without being aware that they are technically breaking their fast because their supplements are not calorie-free. Even branched-chain amino acids (or BCAAS) contain calories, which makes sense considering that some people actually use these for energy during a workout. So here is a tip: it is okay to take supplements and vitamins before or after a fast, but they should generally be avoided during your fasting window. If you do not, then you really are not fasting.

Tip 9. Do not add creams or sweeteners to drinks you are consuming during your fast (such as coffee); you also should not use artificial sweeteners like those contained in diet sodas.

Tip 10. Tea will not break a fast so drink lots of green tea (which will cause you to feel satiated).

Tea is another one of those products that have tons of questions surrounding it when it comes to fasting. Does tea break your fast? Although some choose to avoid tea and anything else substantive like this during a fast, many fitness experts argue that tea will not break your fast. They argue this because tea does not contain compounds that impact metabolism (specifically, it does not impact insulin causing an insulin spike) so you can drink as much tea as you like and your body will still think you are fasting. Green tea can also help you to feel satiated while you are on your fast.

Chapter 10: Tips to Help You Optimize Autophagy

There are many tips out there that can help you to optimize autophagy and achieve your health and fitness goals. Some of these are things you can do while other tips are items that may help you to keep in mind. Here is a free one: food is not necessarily a bad thing. Eating food will cause you to break a fast as your body has to metabolize that food (which sets off a whole chain of metabolic events), but food can do good things for you two. This food fallacy that says that *all* food is *always* bad: well, this is an idea that you should get out of your thinking as quickly as you can. Below are some other tips that can help you make the most out of your dieting, exercising, and fasting with autophagy.

Tip 1. Educate yourself about autophagy.

The best first thing you can do is to educate yourself on the subject. Rome was not built in a day, and your ideal body and perfect life will not be built in a day (if they ever will be built at all). What you need to do is to learn the most about autophagy so that you can know how to do the rights things and avoid the wrong things. If you have read this far then you have already taken an important step in that direction. Here is an opportunity for us to push you on towards continuing that journey.

Tip 2. Ease your way into your new lifestyle.

One of the worst things you can do in any dieting or exercise regimen is to be overambitious. This is not to say that ambition is bad - it certainly is not – but being too ambitious can lead you to be a little unrealistic about what you can accomplish early on in your dieting adventure. If you are used to eating more than 2000 calories a day and consuming lots of sugary drinks as well as other sources of carbohydrates then it will be quite an adjustment for you to do fasting, intermittent fasting, ketogenic diet, or even exercise programs like those involving HIIT. The best thing you can do for yourself is to ease your way slowly into your new lifestyle rather than jump in headfirst.

Tip 3. Incorporate autophagy-stimulating foods into your fasts and diets.

There is a reason why an entire chapter of *Autophagy: Discover How to Live Healthy and Longer with Your Self-Cleansing Body's Natural Intelligence* is devoted to foods that you can eat. Food is one of the best ways that you can stimulate autophagy because everyone needs to eat. You may even find that you like the sorts of foods that are part of your new dieting regimen.

Tip 4. Make a habit of calculating the calories in your foods.

This one is a biggie. Some men and women are already in the habit of tracking the calories in all the foods that they eat. For others, this is a practice that seems unrealistic: one that they will never be able to incorporate into their lives. Keep in mind that you need to start somewhere. If you do not keep track of calories already, you can start by making a habit of reading the labels on all of the foods that you purchase. Those labels are there for a reason. When you realize how unhealthy some of the food that you eat is you may find that you no longer have a desire to eat it (and that is often a good thing).

Tip 5. Make a habit of paying attention to the macronutrient composition of your foods.

Once you have started reading labels you can begin to understand what they mean. The labels on your food not only tell you how many calories are in your food, but they break down your calories by macronutrients. Proteins and carbohydrates have four calories per gram of weight while fat has nine calories per gram. This is why fat slows down your digestion. Your labels also give you a general idea of how much of each macronutrient you should get in the day and how much that particular food is giving you out of that total. These recommendations from the FDA are pretty liberal, but understanding them is an early step in getting the most out of autophagy.

Tip 6. Start eating healthier (less processed) foods.

Once you have started to feel the changes that come from fasting, dieting, and exercise you will be motivated to make other changes in your life. Although this book has not spent a lot of time talking about processed foods, one of the goals of *Autophagy: Discover How to Live Healthy and Longer with Your Self-Cleansing Body's Natural Intelligence* is to help you realize how the things you do are tied to your body's underlying (and natural processes). Most of you will be motivated to continue being healthy and eating less processed food is a huge step in the right direction in terms of bettering your metabolism.

Tip 7. Start buying foods from farmer's markets and local sellers rather than bigger chains.

For some people, the question becomes how you can begin to eat healthier when it feels like everything around you is unhealthy. If you recognize this situation, then you are being very perceptive. Most people in the Western world are inundated with toxic food choices and many people do not have the willpower to resist the temptation to eat unhealthily. An easy way to fix this problem is to surround yourself with healthy food, like those found at your local farmer's market.

Tip 8. Incorporate food timing into your dieting, fasting, and exercise schemes.

Food timing is big in the health and fitness industry. One of the most obvious examples of this is the popularity of oatmeal. Many in the industry advise eating oatmeal in the morning. The reason for this is that oatmeal is a type of complex carb that increases your metabolism. A high metabolism puts your body in fat-burning mode throughout the day. As a slow metabolism is common in obesity-plagued populations, like those in the United States, paying attention to food content and timing can be an easy way to get the most out of autophagy.

Tip 9. Be realistic about what you will and will not be able to accomplish on a diet.

Diets fail for a number of reasons, but one of the big ones is that dieters are not realistic about their diets. In other words, a new dieter will plan to eat 500 calories a day for five days not realizing how little this is in terms of food and that it is unlikely they will stick to this diet. Be realistic. Perhaps you can start at 1000 or 1500 calories a day and work your way to 500 (or whatever your particular dieting goal is).

Tip 10. Combine exercise, fasting, and dieting to help you optimize results.

The best way to optimize autophagy is to combine the three main mechanisms of this pathway into one new lifestyle. Instead of deciding whether or not you want to fast, exercise, or diet, how about you do all three? This is not a hard thing to do. An intermittent fasting diet that involves exercising multiple times a week will accomplish all of this for you.

Glossary

6-Shogoal - the most common of a group of chemicals found in ginger known as shogaols. These chemicals are similar in structure to gingerol. 6-shogaol has been shown to induce autophagy in cancer cells, but not apoptotic cell death.

AMP Kinase - AMP-activated protein kinase is an important enzyme that plays multiple roles in the body, including fatty acid absorption, glucose activation, and oxidation. These processes are part of the larger homeostasis or equilibrium that must be maintained in the body both on a macro level and on a molecular level. AMP-activated protein kinase is sometimes referred to as AMP Kinase or abbreviated as AMPK. AMP Kinase is important in autophagy, and many of the stimulators of autophagy involve activation or increasing concentration of AMP Kinase.

Apoptosis - pre-programmed cell death. Apoptosis is believed to be regulated by a series of triggers or thresholds that stimulate cells and tissues to initiate the process of cell death. Apoptosis, or programmed cell death, should be distinguished from non-programmed (or non-apoptotic) cell death, of which the most pressing example is autophagy.

Atg - autophagy-related genes, of which at least 32 are known.

ATP - Adenosine triphosphate, or ATP, is the major energy molecule found in human beings and most other animals. ATP also plays an important role in homeostasis because of the effect that its breakdown and components have in body tissues like the muscles and liver.

Autophagy - a type of non-apoptotic cell death that is regulated by a variety of genes, proteins, and signaling molecules. The name originates from the Greek and it refers to "self-eating." Autophagy is part of the body's normal process of removing components that are superfluous or non-functional, which makes it distinct from the programmed cell death of apoptosis. Autophagy occurs on a cellular and molecular level through the work of proteins, enzymes, and cellular organelles such as the lysosome.

Cell Death - the general name for the process of destruction of a cell or cellular components. Cell death in the human body is usually divided into apoptotic and non-apoptotic cell death. Autophagy is a type of non-apoptotic cell death, which indicates that though it is carefully regulated it is not programmed in the same manner that apoptosis is.

Chaperone-mediated Autophagy - In this pathway, particles designated for destruction are tagged with a molecule known as a chaperone. The chaperone is there to tag along, alerting the cell's organelles (particularly the lysosome), that this particle is intended for destruction. The particle with the chaperone is recognized by receptors on the lysosomal membrane, which then invaginates the chaperone-tagged particle.

Dry Fasting - the informal name for fasting that is not water fasting.

EGCG - Epigallocatechin gallate, or EGCG, is a catechin found in teas. It is a polyphenol and the most abundant catechin found in tea. Also found in other foods, EGCG has been actively researched because of its potential health benefits. It stimulates autophagy in hepatic cells leading to lipid breakdown. It accomplishes this by increasing the concentration of AMP-activated protein kinase.

Fasting Mimicking Diet - a diet that involves devoting five days out of a 30-day period to a low carbohydrate diet similar to what is seen in the Ketogenic diet. The idea is to "mimic fasting" by shifting the body into Keto during that period so you would basically reap the benefits of a five-day fast even though you actually were eating. During this period, autophagy is used to mobilize fat in hepatic cells and other fat storage areas.

HGH - human growth hormone. Human growth hormone is important in bone and organ growth, health and vivacity, and anti-aging. Human growth hormone levels can be increased by fasting, but these effects are only seen in longer periods of fasting.

HIIT - High-intensity interval training. High-intensity interval training has been shown to improve autophagy. High-intensity interval training uses autophagy to stimulate lipolysis (burning of fat).

Intermittent Fasting - a dieting regimen that involves incorporating periods of fasting into your eating schedule. The most common form of intermittent fasting today is a time-limited program in which the day is broken up into periods of fasting and periods of eating. The schedule is divided into hours of fasting and hours of eating. For example, a 16/8 schedule would mean 16 hours of fasting in the day and 8 hours of eating. Most intermittent fasters choose an eating window, such as 12 noon to 8 PM, that works with their commitments and allow them to easily keep track of when they should be fasting and when they are allowed to eat.

Ketogenic Diet - a diet that involves consuming foods that are extremely low in carbohydrates (or have none), which leads to the production of ketone bodies in the liver. The three ketone bodies produced in the liver are acetoacetate, beta-hydroxybutyrate, and acetone. These ketone bodies can be broken down into a molecule called acetyl-CoA and used as a food source. Ketone bodies are known for their characteristic smell, which has been described as fruity.

Ketone Bodies - the name for three bodies produced by the liver when the body has entered "ketosis" as a result of fasting, starvation, disease process, or other conditions. The three ketone bodies produced by the liver are acetoacetate, beta-hydroxybutyrate, and acetone. These are broken down into a molecule called acetyl-CoA and used as energy.

Ketosis - the state of production of ketone bodies in the liver that typically results from long periods of food deprivation as occurs in fasting or starvation. Ketosis involves autophagy, and many diets like the Ketogenic diet have the explicit goal of inducing ketosis. Ketosis is controversial because although this state has some health benefits, it also can result in poor health outcomes if prolonged or associated with a serious condition, such as diabetes mellitus.

LDL - low-density lipoprotein.

Lysosome - an organelle in the cell that is involved in autophagy through phagocytosis. This organelle works in tandem with other cell organelles, such as the endoplasmic reticulum and the mitochondria to accomplish breakdown of cellular components both as a part of autophagy and outside of it.

Macroautophagy - a process that operates via several steps to trap components in the cytoplasm and recycle them. The first step is the formation of a structure called the isolation membrane. The formation of this structure is triggered by specific factors, some of which will be discussed further shortly. This structure is formed within the cell's cytoplasm; that is, the "sea" of fluid within the cell, as opposed to extracellular fluid outside the cell membrane. Cells are very good at using membranes to separate extracellular components from intracellular ones. This is a means of regulating what is able to enter the cell and protecting the cell.

The second step after the formation of the isolation membrane is the formation of a structure known as the phagophore: a larger structure compared to the initial isolation membrane. The phagophore undergoes a process of expansion which leads to the engulfing of components in the cytoplasm and the formation of a third structure, the autophagosome. The autophagosome may be thought of as the basic essential structure of autophagy. This structure moves towards an important organelle called the lysosome, which results in the fusing of the autophagosome with the lysosome. The result is that the contents of the autophagosome are dumped into the lumen of the lysosome for degradation and recycling.

Macroautophagy is controlled in a highly nuanced manner by a series of triggers. Many of these triggers are in turn signaled and regulated by a number of proteins encoded in genes. Autophagy-related genes, or Atg, refer to proteins involved in the steps that lead to the formation of the autophagosome (via elongation). Triggers of macroautophagy include fasting or starvation, lack of oxygen in the lungs, presence of reactive oxygen species, presence of infectious agents, and therapeutic agents or drugs.

Microautophagy - In microautophagy, the lysosome is the main actor, directly engulfing the components in the cytosol that are intended for degradation. This process involves the double membrane of the lysosome folding in around the components that are being brought into the organelle, a process known as invagination. Like macroautophagy, this process is stimulated by specific triggers, including various environmental factors

OMAD - one meal a day. Essentially an intermittent fasting diet that involves fasting for 23 hours and eating for one hour a day.

Other variations include eating one meal a day every other day, an even longer type of intermittent fasting split.

Phagocytosis - the process of consumption of cell particles, foreign organisms, and debris by lysosomes. Phagocytosis comes from Greek and means "cell eating." It literally refers to the process by which lysosomes, important organelles in the cell, consume and breakdown components with the aid of other organelles, such as the endoplasmic reticulum. This process is generally carefully regulated in the cell with the aid of signaling molecules.

Prebiotic Fiber - foods high in fibers that encourage the growth and maintenance of gut flora. Gut flora is normal bacteria in our GI tract that help us break down food. Examples of prebiotic fiber include artichokes, asparagus, bok choy, and other similar vegetables.

Telomere Effect - the anti-aging effect that can result from fasting. Increasing telomere length can extend the lifetime of our cells and lead to anti-aging benefits.

Water Fasting - an eating regimen that involves supplanting water for food. So the individual will drink quantities of water as part of their fast.

Frequently Asked Questions

1. What is Autophagy and why is it important?

Autophagy refers to the process by which the body degrades and recycles cellular components. Autophagy the term comes from the Greek and it refers to "self-eating." The recycled components can be used as energy. Autophagy can be thought of as a sort of survival of the fittest that occurs on a molecular and cellular level. Cells that are not up to a certain standard are degraded and the components can be used to make new cells. Therefore autophagy can be thought of as important in helping the body achieve a positive balance or homeostasis.

Autophagy is triggered by a number of set factors, including starvation or fasting, lack of oxygen, and the presence of damaging agents such as infectious particles, reactive oxygen species, and others. Autophagy is a form of non-apoptotic cell death, which means that it is not programmed. This does not mean that autophagy occurs haphazardly. Autophagy is triggered and regulated in a highly nuanced way. Factors that stimulate autophagy are always in play as our factors that inhibit it. This allows the right balance to be stuck in a particular tissue.

2. How can I make autophagy work for me?

Most readers are interested in improving their health in one way or another. Autophagy is a natural process that can be tapped into in order to cause dramatic changes in a completely balanced and healthy way. Some people are interested in weight loss and fat loss while others are interested in prolonging their life or improving their quality of life. Autophagy can be used for weight loss because it is the primary tool for lipolysis (fat breakdown) in hepatic tissue and other areas. This means that the best way for you to mobilize fat is to find ways to stimulate autophagy.

But the uses of autophagy extend far beyond weight loss. Much research in the last two decades has focused on how autophagy can be used in specific ways, like to fight cancer. Scientists are in the process of developing targeted therapies that operate by interacting with the body's pathway of autophagy. Some of these therapies stimulate autophagy while others inhibit them. In the case of cancer, stimulating autophagy can remove cells before they become cancerous. Inhibiting autophagy in cells that are already cancerous can push them into apoptosis.

3. Is autophagy different from apoptosis? If so, how?

Apoptosis is programmed cell death. Like autophagy, apoptosis is triggered by a number of factors that the body uses to determine when a cell is no longer needed. In this case, programed just means that once the trigger has been set off, the cell goes through stages of cell death as part of a programmed pathway. Apoptosis is distinct from autophagy in that apoptosis occurs in cells and tissues that cannot be salvaged, and it is associated with death rather than recycling. Apoptosis is almost a self-destruct switch as in a science fiction movie. Autophagy is different. This is a non-programmed cell death that is designed to improve the overall function of the organism.

4. **Is autophagy safe?**

Autophagy is safe because it is a natural process that is constantly occurring in your body. Autophagy allows the body to streamline its cell complement and improve its functioning without having to resort to apoptosis. Autophagy is a process that allows the body to breakdown cells and uses them for energy. In a way, the body feeds on itself in order to be the most ordered, streamline machine that it can be. You should always consult your doctor before beginning any dieting regimen, but you can rest assured that autophagy is entirely safe for you.

Indeed, research has not only found that autophagy is safe but stimulating it is beneficial. The benefits of autophagy are numerous enough that papers detailing them are constantly being published. When it comes to safety, the issues are less of autophagy in general and more concerns about fasting. There are certain medical conditions where fasting can be problematic. Diabetes types 1 and 2 and pregnancy stand out as notable ones. So while autophagy itself is completely safe and natural, some may want to avoid prolonged fasting as a means of stimulating autophagy.

5. Are there any benefits to Autophagy aside from dieting?

Many people who learn about autophagy do so because they are interested in shedding pounds and improving their appearance. But the benefits of autophagy extend far beyond the mere desire to fit into a smaller jean size. Autophagy has been shown to increase longevity, fight cancer, prevent cancer, improve immune function, improve metabolism, improve nervous system functioning, stimulate the release of human growth hormone, and the list goes on. Autophagy is able to do this by having general roles in all cell types, but also by acting in specific ways in specific tissues. For example, autophagy is responsible for the fat breakdown in hepatic cells (lipolysis).

6. Why does autophagy exist?

Autophagy exists because it works. Autophagy is a means for our body to repair damaged tissues, cells, or cellular components without having to resort to programmed cell death or apoptosis. Autophagy is non-programmed or non-apoptotic cell death. Apoptosis should be regarded as a last resort. Programmed cell death is what our body must turn to when its components are beyond the point of salvation. Before this point, some cells and tissues are capable of being repaired and salvaged. In fact, the problem is often an individual cell or an individual protein rather than a damaged area.

The problem may just be that these areas have been exposed to an infectious agent, free radical, or other factors of ultimately external origin. If the body can remove this bad component then it can restore its function and improve it by removing a weak link in the long chain. Remember that these broken down components are then used to build new ones. This should make obvious the underlying benefits of this process to a complicated organism like a human being.

7. Are there different types of autophagy?

There are three major types of autophagy in addition to a large number of subtypes. Autophagy is divided into types based on its mechanism of action. In other words, how autophagy is able to degrade and recycle components. The major types of autophagy are macroautophagy, microautophagy, and chaperone-mediated autophagy (or CMA). Macroautophagy is regarded by some scientists as the most important type. All three involve complex interactions of organelles within the cell.

Macroautophagy occurs via the action of a structure called the autophagosome. This is a double membrane structure that eventually fuses with the lysosome, dumping its contents into it. The autophagosome is formed in stages, beginning with a structure called the isolation membrane. Microautophagy involves primarily the lysosome, which engulfs cellular components by invagination. The third major type of autophagy is chaperone-mediated autophagy. In this type, a molecule marked for degradation is tagged by another molecule called a chaperone. This chaperone is recognized by the lysosome which then degrades the targeted component.

8. Do I have to fast in order to stimulate autophagy?

You do not have to fast in order to stimulate autophagy. Indeed, one of the great things about autophagy is that it can be stimulated in several major ways. Indeed, this picture is so nuanced and complex that one can actually make autophagy work better by incorporating all three major ways of triggering autophagy in your life. The three major ways to stimulate autophagy are through fasting, dieting, and exercise.

Fasting is considered the gold standard for autophagy activation. This is because the human body has been designed to operate on occasional periods of fasting, and most of the many benefits of autophagy have been explicitly linked to fasting, The amount of time that is needed to fast is not set with some choosing to fast for less than 16 hours in a day. It has been suggested however that the ideal fast is between 18 to 24 hours (at least). This type of fast has been shown to be effective at clearing cancer cells from the body. But autophagy can also be stimulated well by diet and exercise. Indeed, both intermittent fasting and the Ketogenic diet have been shown to work well with exercise to trigger powerful autophagy.

9. **Is intermittent fasting a "type" of autophagy?**

Intermittent fasting is basically a stimulator of autophagy rather than a "type" of autophagy. Intermittent fasting is interesting because it is both a type of fasting and a type of diet. Intermittent fasting can involve fasting for an entire day or for a portion of the day. Fasting for a portion of the day is known as time-restricted eating or feeding, and it would involve only eating in a particular window, say, an eight-hour period, and then fasting for the rest of the day. Intermittent fasting has been shown to work well with an exercise program, such as a HIIT program, although it can also be used as a standalone trigger for autophagy.

10. Is it safe to do intermittent fasting or other types of fasting to stimulate autophagy if I am diabetic or have another serious health condition?

You should always consult a doctor before starting in any health, fitness, or dieting program. This is especially true if you have health problems that require you to take medication. Although human beings have been fasting for hundreds of thousands of years and fasting has been shown to be healthy in most people, there are some cases in which this type of diet may be contraindicated. Many diabetics are able to intermittently fast, but because they have to monitor their blood sugar it may be necessary to either have a generous eating window or to be prepared to break their fast if necessary. Intermittent fasting, however, would certainly be safer than the Ketogenic diet, which would be contraindicated in diabetics.

11. Are there any advantages to intermittent fasting compared to other types of diets that are based on autophagy?

One of the main benefits of intermittent fasting is that, if you do the time-restricted protocol, you are able to incorporate periods of eating into your day rather than fasting for longer periods or even the whole day as you may in other types of diets. This may work better with the schedules of some people. It also works for people that have health problems that making fasting difficult or flat-out contraindicated. There are other benefits to the intermittent fasting diet as well. These have been specifically shown to be found in intermittent fasting although some of these benefits overlap with the overall autophagy benefits. Some of these benefits include improved fat loss, improved cardiovascular functioning, improved glucose control, increased lifespan, reduced muscle loss, reduced hunger, improved metabolism, improved self-image and energy, reduced risk of cancer, and reduced risk of neurodegenerative disease (among others).

12. **What are the best foods for me to eat if I am trying to stimulate autophagy?**

This is one of the most popular questions that people ask when it comes to autophagy. Many foods stimulate autophagy, but the so-called big four are ginger, green tea, reishi mushrooms, and turmeric/curcumin. These foods are all important in the Ayurvedic Medicine of Asia.

Research has shown that their health benefits are so numerous that it is difficult to list them. Many if not most of these benefits can be attributed to their ability to stimulate autophagy in specific cells in the body. These foods generally have anti-cancer benefits, anti-aging benefits, and positive metabolic properties.

13. Is it true that autophagy can help fight cancer?

It has been shown that stimulating autophagy can be effective in treating and preventing several types of cancer, especially colon cancer and lung cancer. This is a general benefit of autophagy stimulation as well as a specific benefit of some stimulators, such as some types of food (see the chapter on foods that stimulate autophagy). Autophagy helps to fight cancer both by triggering cell death in cells before they become cancerous and by helping degrade cancer cells.

14. How should I decide what type of diet I should go on?

Many factors go into the decision of choosing the best diet for you. Many men and women make this decision based on their specific weight loss goals. For example, someone attempting to lose weight quickly might decide to resort to diets that claim to cause dramatic weight loss, like the paleo diet or Atkins diet. In this book, we review diets that trigger autophagy: namely the Ketogenic diet, intermittent fasting, water fasting, and fasting-mimicking diet. The big difference between these diets is how restrictive they are in terms of when you can eat (and to a lesser extent, how much you eat). For most people considering autophagy, the question becomes whether they are healthy enough to withstand a long fast. Some people like to start out with fasting-mimicking diet or water fast rather than jump into a more restrictive type of intermittent fasting diet or Keto.

15. What is fasting-mimicking, and are there any benefits to this type of diet compared to some of the others?

The Fasting Mimicking Diet bears some similarities to other diets in that it closely follows caloric intake and macronutrients. This diet allows dieters interested in reaping the benefits of diets like the Ketogenic diet or intermittent fasting to tap into these without many of the restrictions. The Fasting Mimicking Diet devotes five days out of a 30-day period to caloric restriction similar to what is seen in Keto while the remaining 25 days are less restrictive. The idea here is to trick the body into thinking it is starving. In this situation, the body will mobilize adipose (fat) stores for energy rather than circulating sugar.

16. How often should I fast?

This is a common question for those interested in integrating fasting into their lifestyle and dieting regimens because of the numerous benefits. The answer to this question is that it varies based on age. Some health and fitness gurus argue that it is better for those over the age of 40 to modify traditional intermittent fasting regimens because a slower metabolism with age leads them to benefit more from a modification.

Specifically, those over the age of 40 can benefit from a normal day of eating (i.e. without any intermittent fasting) followed by a longer than normal period of fasting, such as 20 hours. A typical intermittent fasting regimen is 16 hours of fasting and 8 hours of eating in a 24 hour period. In this example, someone over the age of 40 would have a 20 hour period of fasting punctuated by days of normal eating before and after (therefore fasting every other day). This not only allows them to benefit even more greatly from the anti-aging effects of fasting (such as the telomere effect) because of the longer fasting period, but it also allows them to incorporate their altered metabolism into their dieting regimen better. For those under 40, a traditional 16/8 intermittent fasting schedule can work if intermittent fasting is the road you intend to take.

17. Are there any health benefits to fasting for longer periods?

There are. In fact, research has suggested that the greatest impact of autophagy comes when men and women fast for longer periods (at least 18 hours). Indeed, some studies suggest that fasting for even longer periods, as happens in some cultural and religious groups; the anti-aging and anti-cancer effects are even greater. Although greater information is needed for these benefits to be more clearly delineated and understood, some choose to integrate longer periods of fasting one or two times a year into their general regimen of intermittent fasting or water fasting.

18. Can I drink caffeine when I am fasting?

Some recommend avoiding caffeine altogether during a fast. Others argue that caffeine should be avoided because of some of its stimulating effects, but is not prohibited. The general answer is that you can consume this during your fast, although the recommendation is that if you are going to drink caffeine that you should have it earlier in the day. It has been suggested that caffeine throughout the day may be acceptable in younger people, but can cause problems in older individuals. The issues center on catecholamines like adrenaline that is stimulated by caffeine. Stimulating these catecholamines throughout the day can lead to a type of fatigue called adrenal fatigue that can leave you feeling tired and worse for wear. So if you do need your coffee and tea during your days of fasting, make sure you do it earlier in the day.

19. Can I take supplements and vitamins while I am fasting?

The general consensus here is that you should avoid vitamins and supplements altogether during a fast. There are several reasons for this, but a major one is that vitamins and anti-oxidants can screw with your metabolism and therefore undue the autophagy effects of the fast.

20. Are there any recommendations for breaking a fast?

The general recommendation is to focus on foods that are high in protein and fiber. In an abstract sense, this type of diet is what our human bodies expect us to be eating and therefore not only are less of a shock to the system (compared to highly processed foods and grains) but also help us in terms of getting our GI system moving in a positive way. The recommendation for a first meal is 25% of your body weight in grams of protein (so about 42 grams of protein for a 150 lb. individual). Also, a meal high in prebiotic fiber to get the gut flora back to normal is also a good idea. Prebiotic fiber includes things like asparagus, artichoke, and bok choy.

21. Are there any benefits to the Ketogenic diet?

Fasting is regarded as the be-all and end-all when it comes to stimulating autophagy, but dieting and exercise are extremely powerful, and many people live long, healthy lives without having to fast at all (although many people actually "fast" without doing it consciously.

The Ketogenic diet has become very popular very quickly because of the dramatic effects it can have on your body. Many people have gone from obese size to a normal BMI with the Ketogenic diet. The benefits of the Ketogenic diet include a reduction in blood glucose, increase in insulin sensitivity (and reduced insulin levels), improved organ functioning, improved concentration, lower triglyceride levels, lower blood pressure, and lower blood sugar.

22. What are the best ways to induce autophagy?

Autophagy can be induced or stimulated in a variety of ways. Fasting is one of the most reliable ways of stimulating autophagy, and it is recommended by health enthusiasts who have actively studied the best ways to activate this pathway. Fasting can take a variety of forms, including the well-known intermittent fasting, or so-called alternate day fasting, which involves punctuating days of fasting with "normal" days of eating. Dieting and exercise can also be used to predictably stimulate autophagy. The main ways of stimulating this pathway (that will be examined here) include:

- Fasting
- Dieting with the Ketogenic Diet (or similar regimens)
- Exercise, especially HIIT (high-intensity interval training)

23. Are there other types of autophagy that it is useful to know about?

There are several other types of autophagy that have been studied in addition to the main three types. Some of these fall under the three categories of macroautophagy, microautophagy, and chaperone-mediated autophagy, while others can be regarded as standalone pathways. For example, aggrephagy is regarded as a type of macroautophagy. Some lesser-known types of autophagy include.

Zymography: the detection and degradation of granules in the pancreas

Xenography: the degradation of toxic and infectious particles

Ribophagy: the breakdown of ribosomes

Pexography: the breakdown of peroxisomes (a type of organelle)

Aggrephagy: the degradation of cellular protein aggregates in macroautophagy

Conclusion

Autophagy evolved to help you be the streamlined machine that you ought to be. This process aids the body by helping it to degrade components, such as cells, that do not meet the body's high standards and expectations. Autophagy prevents waste by allowing the body to remove components that detract from core functions. Cellular components that are broken down can be reused to build new cells and also can be used for energy.

Indeed, lipolysis in hepatic cells and other areas where adipose tissue is formed represents one of the aspects of autophagy that is of most benefit to those looking to tap into this cellular process. Naturally, this is because many people looking to utilize autophagy are trying to burn fat and lose weight, but it is also because fat breakdown and metabolism represent a major step in the right direction towards improving your health.

In ***Autophagy:*** *Discover How to Live Healthy and Longer with Your Self-Cleansing Body's Natural Intelligence,* you learned how you can tap into autophagy to achieve a variety of metabolic goals. Autophagy has become quite popular in recent years, but it is easy to get lost in the quagmire of figuring out what precisely it is how to use it. Indeed, as you have seen, autophagy underlies many of the popular diets and therapies that can change your life, including cancer drugs that are being developed as we speak.

In the first chapter, you began your forays into Autophagy and stimulating it by embarking on an in-depth tour of the subject. You learned that this tool to help you live longer and better is happening constantly within your body as part of your body's survival of the fittest order. Autophagy takes place on a cellular level, and it is triggered by several factors that you can learn to stimulate in order to achieve your health and fitness goals. Indeed, many learn that autophagy is crucial to so many processes in the body that their lives improve dramatically merely by tapping into it one form.

There are many benefits to be gained by tapping into autophagy. These benefits extend beyond the realm of weight loss and fitness. Autophagy has been shown incontrovertibly to be influential in immune functioning, cancer-fighting, metabolism, and longevity. Learning what to do with autophagy begins, in part, by learning what it can do for you. Some of the benefits of autophagy include:

- Improved metabolism and insulin sensitivity
- Improved immune functioning
- Improved DNA repair and stabilization
- Anti-aging effects
- Anti-cancer effects
- Improved exercise tolerance
- Improved cardiovascular function
- Improved nervous system functioning

- Protection from neurodegenerative disease
- Protection from infection
- Improved sense of health and wellness
- Improved quality of life

Autophagy is complex, but that should not dissuade you from using this tool to achieve a better, healthier life. Most people want a life free from disease, filled with positive vibes and energy, where they can enjoy the benefits of being slim and feeling healthy. Autophagy can accomplish this for you, and it does in three ways. The three major types of autophagy – macroautophagy, microautophagy, and chaperone-mediated autophagy – were explored, and you were introduced to some subtypes of this process that are also important and which continue to be actively studied.

Naturally, the autophagy discussion would not be complete if the reader did not learn how they can stimulate it in their own body. Autophagy can be triggered in various ways of which the three most important are fasting, dieting, and exercise. These states trigger the body to begin conserving and streamlining processes, which include removing components that are poorly-functioning or dysfunctional. This can include cells that are not up to snuff, but it can also include cancer cells. Autophagy can also be stimulated in other ways, such as by reduced oxygen as happens in exercise.

Dieting is one of the most popular ways to stimulate the process of autophagy in the human body. The dividing line between dieting and fasting is not always clear as most "fasting" that is done to stimulate autophagy includes a diet of one sort or another. In **Autophagy**: *Discover How to Live Healthy and Longer with Your Self-Cleansing Body's Natural Intelligence,* you learned how water fasting and ketosis diets can be used to stimulate autophagy in powerful ways. Water fasting works because water contains no calories so you are technically fasting while you are drinking it. Ketosis diets like the Ketogenic diet work because they involve placing your body in ketosis, which results in fat stores being mobilized for energy in the form of ketones. This leads to weight loss and other health benefits.

Diets that tap into this metabolic process are perfect for men and women whose goals are focused less on weight loss and more on muscle preservation. Targeted fat loss is just as important to people who are trying to build (and show) their muscle as it is to people who are trying to lose weight. Intermittent fasting is one of the standouts in the world of Autophagy because of its proven success in helping professional athletes, bodybuilders, fitness competitors, and others achieve their personal and professional goals.

Intermittent fasting involves separating periods of eating by fasting. This fasting period can be as long or as short as you want. Some people choose to engage in alternate-day fasting, which involves fasting for 24 hours followed by a day of eating, while others opt for time-restricted feeding in which they break down their day into periods of eating and fasting. The 16/8 protocol, in which 16 hours are spent fasting and eight hours are spent eating in a 24-hour period, is a popular version of this protocol. Intermittent fasting has been attached to a wide variety of health benefits, many of which overlap with the benefits of the process of autophagy as it has been explored in this book.

Foods are a powerful stimulator of metabolic processes in the body. It is not difficult to understand why this is. Your body's basal metabolic rate is altered by your eating behavior. If you eat diets high in carbohydrates, fats, and processed foods, your body's metabolism tends to slow down. If you eat healthier foods that are low in carbs and less processed your metabolic rate rises (which is something that you want). In ***Autophagy: Discover How to Live Healthy and Longer with Your Self-Cleansing Body's Natural Intelligence,*** you learned about three superfoods that you can incorporate into your dieting and exercise regimens. Ginger, green tea, turmeric, and reishi mushrooms have been used consumed for centuries because of their positive health benefits, and it turns out that most of these benefits are tied to autophagy.

Mimicking fasting refers to a type of diet that involves stimulating autophagy by tricking the body into thinking that it is fasting. As you learned, fasting is the gold standard for autophagy stimulation. Research suggests that a 7-day fast may be enough to completely clear cancer cells from the body. The fasting-mimicking diet involves consuming low calories over a period of five days. It also is important to keep close track of your macronutrients. This diet is an option for those who have reservations about fasting or are unable to fast.

Some people learn best by absorbing the tricks of the trade-in convenient lists. In chapters nine and ten, you learned the tips that you can use to help you with fasting and to optimize Autophagy. You were familiarized with some of the important terms mentioned in this book to ensure that you were able to get the most out of the information provided here. Autophagy can change your life. All it will take is a little hard work and education on your end. Oh, and a little green tea every now and again doesn't hurt either.

9 781694 478238